Broad Arrows

A Mystical Walk Through the Land of Enchantment

Anne Westcott

PublishAmerica

Baltimore

ISBN: 1-4241-0338-X
PUBLISHED BY PUBLISHAMERICA, LLLP
www.publishamerica.com
Baltimore

Printed in the United States of America

Here's to my parents,
gentle warriors who have moved on the
happy hunting-ground, finally at rest.

The author wishes to thank:

Tom Kennedy of the Zuni Tourism Department for filling the blanks in my memory, Merla Wilson for feeding my mind and body, Peter Lathwood for his continued confidence in my work.

And special thanks to Ruth Herbert for reading and suggesting changes in the writing of this manuscript.

Chapter 1—The Mother Road

It was the ugliest town I ever saw. Faded ads and weathered store fronts disintegrated my hopes. Suddenly, my future turned bleak.

Looking out the train window at once colorful designs, now dull and faded, I sat anxious and confused, refusing to let the symptoms of culture shock take over my mind completely.

As we passed each washed out notice on the commercial buildings, it felt like I was turning pages of a *Country Gazette* giving the impression the residents here were falling apart like the town; healing oil for barbed wire cuts, toothache gum, a rupture cure, and the likeness of a pallid green frog, looking directly at me, selling nerve pills that read, "Don't Be Nervous."

Rolling into town my hopes crumbled to the ground along with the brick buildings. Here I was, yet again, making another new beginning with total strangers.

Corrugated panels of rust were holding many of the assemblages together with bits of scrap iron, like the whole town had been put together by a tinsmith; a flat plate of a town in dark negative images fast developing a visible picture of my sinking heart. My first train ride was pleasant enough but actually seeing Gallup for the first time was a shock, and my prevailing thought was, "I don't think I can live here."

I sat on the edge of the flattened vinyl cushion thinking I had nothing left to lose. I *had* to give my newfound retreat *calling* a try and this town came with the deal. Three months earlier I had landed in a hospital stricken with multiple sclerosis and could hardly walk or talk. My progress had been encouraging, remarkable really, and I wanted to give this new opportunity a fair chance. I really did have nothing left to lose.

Throughout the trip I monitored my health like a diagnostician as we followed historic Route 66—no numbness as we cruised into San Bernadino; astigmatism in my eyes was holding steady entering

Kingman; nausea completely absent on the heights of Flagstaff; and I had been headache-free all the way into Gallup blazing a trail of soundness of my own along Route 66.

Thank God the train ride hadn't made me nauseous, I thought with relief. Nausea had been the major concern for me in thinking how the side-to-side swaying motion of the train combined with the constant forward sliding of steel on the tracks might affect me. Wasn't this enough to make anyone feel sick? I had learned to never go anywhere now without carrying a few sea sickness pills (antivert); the drug had been a Godsend for me by stopping nausea. One pill before climbing aboard and I was fine during the entire thirteen hour journey.

Before my four day hospital stay, I had spent two years outside of Tucson in one of the strictest monasteries there is, the same order Thomas Merton had joined and wrote voluminiously about (Trappists for men and Trappistines for women; properly called Cistercian). Deciding to leave was the hardest decision of my life, and now with my vocation behind me, I was forced to rejoin the fast-paced secular world. Unable to go back to a slower time, I chose the next best thing, the slower lifestyle in a small town. I chose Gallup.

The question foremost in my mind was, is it possible to practice what I learned in the monastery at a retreat?

The sound of the whistle brought the crew out of the yard in a reluctant trot and as the train approached the station I could see people getting off the benches in a murmured gathering, one woman already crying, another looking as if she was about to, in preparation to embrace and kiss in welcome. As a stranger in a strange land, I was greeted by a familiar knot in the pit of my stomach, fear.

"Gaaallup" I heard the black porter shout loudly in a long drawn-out tone as he walked up and down the aisle, his thin black tie swinging from his white collar as he leaned in close making sure all the passengers knew to get off if this was their destination.

Sure, he could be calm, I thought, he wasn't getting off here.

"Gaaaallup," the cadence announced again, his voice trailing away as he went into a connecting car taking the strong scent of his cologne with him.

After sitting the duration of the train trip, I stood up stiffly. I inched toward the exit, moving my hold from head-rest to head-rest to steady myself and shuffled my way slowly down the crowded aisle toward the open section along with everyone else. Mentally I took stock of my walking-so far I was doing okay. My right leg felt heavy but manageable and I didn't think Sr. Hyacinth could notice any weakened muscle coordination. Only I could.

Because Gallup is a typical Western town, the train was filled with ranchers wearing jeans with bold silver belt buckles and cowboy boots, and Native American women arrayed in silver and turquoise jewelry with beaded necklaces dangling from their necks. And me in my jeans, wearing no jewelry at all, holding tightly onto the cowboy hat I wore in the monastery like a security blanket.

We had pulled in aligned with the platform where I noticed a heavyset Sister, plump as a dumpling, dressed in a knee length black habit and veil searching the handfuls of disembarking passengers for one fitting my description. She didn't have to look hard. I think I was the only blonde on the train.

Stepping off the train I could feel light puffs of a November breeze as I made my way through the crowd. I staggered slightly as I took my first unhindered steps in hours on the strip of cement running alongside the train. My eyes gave it a close sidelong scan as I passed; the degree of controlled power it maintained was exhilarating with its large steel wheels, levers that looked stronger than crowbars, hard rods and powerful engines able to pull tons of cars.

Drawing my eyes from the cowcatcher on the front of the train, I looked over and saw the only person wearing a habit on the platform, maybe in the entire town. This has to be Sr. Hyacinth, I thought with a sudden relief, glad someone actually showed up to collect me. She was standing in the black habit of a Franciscan anxiously searching the crowd of arrivals making their way off the train. Large boned, strong frame, piercing eyes; she looked as intimidating as the train.

I could tell she was a good schmoozer though, making good humored remarks to the others waiting around her. She had the cheery disposition of a Mrs. Claus with rosy cheeks and a jolly nature to match and I liked her happy personality immediately.

I didn't know that much about Franciscans, only they were probably kind to animals because of the reputation of their founder, Saint Francis of Assisi, a friar known for helping animals. It did bring to mind the notion that if I told her about my MS, she might see me as an injured stray, and after my ordeal in the hospital, I certainly felt like a wounded animal.

So pulling my hair back tighter in my beret and straightening my bangs with my fingers, I took a deep breath and stepped in front to face her. But before I had a chance to say anything, she smiled a friendly smile and held out her hand in welcome. Then in a high-pitched voice, puffing forth as powerful and controlled as the whistle on the train, I heard, "Welcome to Indian country."

The pallid green frog painted on the wall selling nerve pills had been right all along, there *was* no reason to nervous.

Chapter 2—The Last Frontier

As we walked to Sister's car I looked around the colorless depot. It seemed to me everything was decaying—from rotted fruit in a crumpled trash can to benches with rusted iron arm rests. Nothing seemed to be broken or falling apart; it wasn't wracked and ruined, just dissolving and wasting away.

The small railway's parking lot was filled with old GMC trucks. Introducing me to Gallup, Sr. Hyacinth told me that in this town GMC stood for Grand Mother's Car. "That's nice," I said politely, not understanding what she meant.

"See there," she said, pointing in the back of a truck as we pulled out into traffic.

"I'll be darned," trying not to stare but feeling my eyes widening in disbelief. "That's the grandmother sitting in the *back* of the truck?"

"That's how it is here. It's customary," Sr. Hyacinth said matter-of-factly. I looked closely as we pulled up behind them at a traffic light. Snuggled into a bed of blankets was indeed an older Navajo woman in a drab scarf covering her head with only her face exposed. And if this was a foretaste of unconventional experiences to come, not only did I need to pull my eyes away, I should set aside my usual way of judging as well. This wasn't LA anymore, this was Gallup. Right then, I made a conscious decision; no matter how unattractive and unappealing this frontier town, I would force myself to *try* to like it.

Sister Hyacinth promptly instructed me never to photograph a person or even a group in this part of the country without asking their permission.

"Really, it's a matter of respect," she said. "You're taking something from them, their image, and many believe is taking their spirit, so we have to respect that."

"Don't worry, I didn't bring my camera," already regretting my decision.

We were driving on a smoothly paved highway speeding up a long steady grade when I saw a dog roaming aimlessly on the next hill. As we passed it, I saw it had bare patches on its wrinkled skin. Homeless and sickly besides convinced me I somehow drew this four-footed mangy mongrel into my vision by our similar situations. Not a nice welcoming committee.

The landscape was brown and colorless, one boring hill running into another, a bland match with the train depot. Sr. Hyacinth was obviously proud of her town offering enthusiastic sightseeing jaunts to take; trading posts, art galleries, Native American dances to see. She was so unlike the silent demeanor of the Cistercians, I thought, but it didn't take me long to get used to this talkative nun, her comments laced with frequent smatterings of laughter.

"Gallup is such a beautiful city, with so many things to see and do, don't you agree?"

"To be honest with you Sister, I really haven't seen much of the town," I answered. "As far as I can tell from the stops the *Southwest Chief* made along the way, trains seem to pull into some of the dumpiest parts of town alongside smashed up and disabled engines waiting for repairs. Entering Gallup wasn't any different. And with the heavy smell of oil and grease hanging thickly in the air when we rolled in, I'd have to say what I've seen of your town is Gallup's back-end," clarifying my opinion.

"Ha, right you are," she snickered, thinking about it and laughing again.

The scruffy brown rabbitbrush with its golden-yellow heads growing along the highway was lost on my attentiveness to how I was feeling, and especially on how good it was going to feel when we finally stopped moving. During the entire train ride I tried to concentrate on things far away to combat motion sickness before it started. My taut muscles told me I was still tensing. Thirteen hours worth.

Sitting next to this likable nun it seemed a shame to spoil her narrated travelogue with my unfavorable picture I had of her town. She was a veritable wealth of information, commenting how Gallup was situated at an elevation of 6,500 feet, and the retreat center was about a thousand feet higher than that.

"Snowfall seldom stays on the ground for more than two or three days at a time, if we *have* snow." She went on, "Gallup winters are cold, but with plenty of sunshine."

"It won't be long now," pointing to the Navajo reservation we were passing on the right. I was surprised it wasn't marked at all, no signs, fences or barricades. Only a few sheep wandering over an adjacent field. I didn't know what I was expecting, maybe a few cow skulls dangling feathers as a warning to those entering. I soon learned Indian reservations looked the same as any other land so a visitor would have to know beforehand they were passing over the boundary line.

"The Zuni reservation is just up the road 26 miles," making the point how the phrase *just up the road* is used often and could mean anything from a mile to hundreds of miles. "Try not to learn the hard way," she laughingly cautioned with a smile.

I pushed off her meaning. Her words, "it wouldn't be long now" had sent a wave of nervousness through me. I was still debating with myself whether I should disclose my recent hospital stay and illness to her. What was the right thing to do? She wouldn't notice my slower gait or my slight eye twitches. She wouldn't know I was still straightening out and unfurling my limbs and trying to walk normally. She didn't know me before MS had crumpled me up like a wad of paper.

Everything about multiple sclerosis was difficult, difficult to spell and pronounce. Why couldn't I have contracted an illness people were somewhat familiar with like consumption, impetigo, or blood poisoning? This difficult disease might actually ruin my chances here before I even got started. I *could* get away with keeping it to myself if I wanted to.

But my time here was more important than being just a job. It was seeing if I fit into a new vocation. How could I start a spiritual way of life by omitting something so important? I couldn't. I decided I would have to tell her at some point.

"Pinon trees, turquoise, and chile peppers. This is the genuine Gallup," Sister announced as we turned off the highway and onto a steep dirt driveway so ribbed it looked like an old wash-board and made her sound like someone was knocking on her Adam's apple when she spoke. "Ja ja ja nuu inn Ga ga aa lup." Hyacinth said again while I held on to the seat. Looking all around me anxiously waiting my first view of the Retreat Center, I was feeling as jittery on the inside as the road was making me feel on the outside. Could I really force myself to stay in a repulsive place if I didn't have the stomach for working in dilapidated buildings that looked worse than the depot? Was this volunteer experience like a lobster trap, easy to get into but hard to get out of?

The roadside banks were overgrown with a variety of weeds fighting for domain growing thicker on the drop-off side of the hill but thinning as we crested. At the top of the driveway we joined a smooth, level, well-maintained road, but still unpaved. Making a hard left, we turned in and I had my first glimpse of the Retreat Center.

It wasn't Cinderella's garden with bluebirds tying bows in the air and squirrels festooning my hair with ribbons, but it wasn't altogether horrible either. Reddish-brown bushy tailed squirrels were scampering about and greedy dive-bombing blue jays were zeroing in at the grape-sized red berries hanging on the shrubs, all without a Disney score.

When Sr. Hyacinth finally turned off the engine and I stepped out, I did feel the tranquil feeling of suspended calm one might expect an enchanted garden to have.

Weeds had taken over for the most part. Walkways looked like flower beds for the heartiest of weeds, growing in and out of low rock borders, making their tangled way up the smooth reddish bark of manzanita branches in undergrowth that was choking the life out of huge sprawling shrubs. Mixed in with this horticultural fray were medium sized juniper trees placed around the periphery of the property for a windbreak, frail with branches depleted of new growth, looking as if they had been blasted by snow, sleet and freezing rain winter after winter.

In between the shrubbery I could see a long building on the left that needed a new coat of redwood paint, and six small irregularly shaped log cabins on the opposite side of the yard that followed the road as it circled around. There was a newer building on the right made out of regular lumber, not logs, painted with a light varnish that had a newness to it in its clean and unmarred state. In the center of the roof was a metal cross, about a yard high, and I knew this was the retreat chapel. And resting heavily in the center of the weeds was a large bell in a wooden frame, the frame needing another coat of redwood paint as well. Scaly rust coated its clapper as it rested on the ground.

I was told the six cabins encircling the yard were for retreatants but they weren't called cabins, they were called *hogans* after the Navajo dwellings in an effort to give guests a sense of Indian authenticity. "We call them white-man hogans because they have running water and electricity unlike on reservation land."

Surprised, I asked, "What, Indian hogans don't have running water?" but from the look of the train depot it shouldn't have surprised me.

"That's right. They have to haul the water in from wells. There is a well here," she said, pointing up over a slope and away from the retreat. "Wells are put on neutral property such as church property, I think, so it won't cause any friction among the tribes. Either that or they can't afford to hire people to do the drilling. You'll hear the trucks. They ramble up the driveway at all hours with large empty barrels in the back so they can fill them with water. This is one of the reasons the driveway is in the shape it's in. It gets plenty of use."

"In this day and age," I commented but afraid to ask if the Retreat worked in the same way.

As soon as we stopped, I opened the car door and stretched. It felt good to move after the hours of sitting. And it felt good to fill my lungs with deep breaths of clean pine-filled air.

Talking as we walked to the front door, Sr. Hyacinth continued explaining the design of the complex. "Each of our hogans were built with a skylight dome in the center of the roof like authentic hogans in keeping with their notion of letting the bad spirits out while keeping good spirits in, but letting the smoke from their fire out as well. Our sky holes are covered with hard clear plastic, while Navajo hogans are not. A hole in the roof could be a problem during rain and snow," Sr. Hyacinth said, squinting as she thought about the damage these scenarios could bring. "But unlike authentic hogans built with their entrance facing east to welcome the sun like traditional Navajo dwellings, our hogans were designed to fit the curvature of the road. It's hard to see because of the weeds but this road circles around by each hogan for unloading of luggage by retreatants."

The little I knew about retreat work, I thought the Retreat should at least look presentable. As it was, all that was missing was a for-sale sign posted out in front alerting prospective buyers. I thought clearing the road would be a good place for me to start.

Unlocking the door of a large building, Sr. Hyacinth led the way into a hallway and passing two offices told me the front part of the building was for administration and the back part was used as a convent where she stayed. "You'll stay in *Brother Sun's* hogan. Each hogan has been named after a different feature from a poem by our founder, St. Francis. There is *Brother Sun, Sister Moon, Brother Wind, Sister Water, Brother Fire*, and our largest hogan we named *Sister Mother Earth*. I hope you won't mind being separated from the main house, but you'll be comfortable."

I wasn't worried about comfort, I was thinking about my safety and about being over there by myself. "Is there a phone?" I asked, my question unheard as we walked through the Retreat.

"Here, of course, is the kitchen," as we entered a spacious work area as clean as an operating room. It was what I would expect in a restaurant; a large hood over the stove, butcher block counters, professional mixers, coffee makers, and stainless steel serving containers. As I passed the two large sinks I quickly turned on a faucet. Clean cool water squirted out. Good, no traipsing to the well with barrels for water.

"This is a good kitchen," I told her, like I knew what I was talking about, pretending the equipment met with my approval. The kitchen could have been equipped an egg-beater and a bowl for all I knew about Retreat kitchens.

"Credit Sr. Celeste, the other Franciscan Sister assigned to Gallup with me. She's French and does an excellent job of it. She does all the cooking when we have a retreat on, but during the week she supervises a home for girls in town. Sometimes she starts a meal at the home and adds the finishing touches here. A literal 'meals on wheels' production at times."

And opening a door from the kitchen, Sr. Hyacinth took a dramatic step back out of the way so I could have my first unobstructed look and said, "Welcome to St. Francis Retreat."

I felt my eyebrows involuntarily raise and mouth went slack, hanging open like my jaw unhinged. It was the most beautiful room I ever saw! If it wasn't Cinderella's garden out in front, this palatial room could have been her ballroom. Smooth lengths of redwood formed three long arches on the ceiling that extended the entire width of the room, from the kitchen wall to the opposite window. The rest of the roof was finished in great redwood planks tingeing the entire room with the soft red color of the wood. The natural wood decor was magnificent.

Stepping into this room was like stepping into a glare of heaven. This great room felt like a cathedral with its structural characteristics inspiring spiritual insights. But this timeless statement of faith wasn't built around hand-carved limestone carvings or a gothic style architecture. It was done by simply letting the beauty of the landscape grace the room naturally by surrounding the room with three sides of windows. At one point I thought I heard a distant choir.

At the other end of the room was a huge stone fireplace and hearth and it crossed my mind that it may have been put together by an Indian craftsman, with their penchant for design in weaving rugs and blankets. A wooden crucifix with corpse hung on the fireplace big enough to be seen by an entire dining room filled with retreatants. And on both sides of the fireplace were two large windows made up of many smaller square windows, twenty-five windows on each side. The rug, which was a pale shade of burnt orange, connected the ceiling to the floor in color, the striking color of the room enveloping everything. Ten round walnut-grained tables finished the dining room with low-backed chairs pulled in close to each table.

Walking the length of the dining room under the high graceful arches, we angled around the tables as we made our way toward the bright reflection of light at the other end. I followed Sr. Hyacinth as we passed the dining section and entered an area used for conferences. A long couch had been placed in front of the fireplace with many throw pillows on top of it. Extra stacks of chairs had been pulled off to the side flanked it. This beautiful room was the working hub of the Retreat Center.

Reaching the massive fireplace, Hyacinth stopped. Stepping out from behind her, I raised my eyes to follow her gaze and did a double take. Below us was a great expanse of reservation land that went on for centuries, the late afternoon sun emblazoning the entire landscape in golden incandescence, the clouds shimmering with bright gilded edges.

"Beauty before me, beauty behind me, beauty above me, beauty beneath me," Sr. Hyacinth spoke softly, as we scanned the endless sky together; the view acting better than a drug still my nervousness. "That's a Navajo prayer," and without turning to face me, neither of us wanting take our eyes off the breathtaking view, in a motionless calm asked, "Is there any place more beautiful than Gallup?"

I thought for a moment as I admired the lacing of soft vistas, the majestic rock formations, and the empty plain I was gazing over combined with Indian lore, all of which filled me with wonder and decisively answered, "No, I can't say I've ever seen a more beautiful place than Gallup."

Chapter 3—Praises of Creatures

I have never slept in anything resembling a hogan before, even a modernized version, and the prospect of doing so left my imagination in a lively state. I expected to see a bear skin rug near the entrance complete with furry head, glass eyes, and yellowed teeth as a ferocious reminder of what *could* crawl in if the skyhole wasn't covered; anything that will keep out snarling and growling I was all for.

Instead, when Sr. Hyacinth turned the key in the lock of the undersized door of the hogan marked "Brother Sun," I was face to face with a creature of a tamer nature, for hanging on a wall close to the front door was a picture of the founder of the Franciscan order next to a copy of his poem:

> Praise be to thee, my lord, with all Thy creatures. Especially to my worshipful Brother Sun, which lights up the day and through him dost Thou brightness give, and beautiful is he and radiant with splendor great.
>
> Praised be to my Lord for Sister Moon and for the Stars in heaven. Thou hast formed them clear and precious and fair. Praised be my Lord for Brother Wind, and for the air and clouds and fair and every kind of weather by which Thou givest to Thy creatures nourishment.
>
> Praised be my Lord for Sister Water, which is greatly helpful and humble and precious and pure.
>
> Praised be to my Lord for Brother Fire, by which Thou lighted up the dark; and fair is he and gay and mighty and strong.
>
> Praised be to my Lord for our Sister Mother Earth, which sustains and keeps us and brings forth fruits, grass, and flowers bright.

Praise be to my Lord for our Sister Death, from which
no living man can flee. Woe to them, who die in mortal sin;
blessed those who find themselves in Thy most holy will.
St. Francis of Assisi

"There's one in every hogan," Sister said, not losing sight as to why
she was stationed here in the first place, and I thought it was a good
thing there were only five hogans because I didn't think many people
would want to sleep in a Sister Death hogan.

The eight-sided hogan was bathed in light, and stepping under the
skyhole I threw my head as far back as it would go and stared upward.
I marveled at the blue New Mexico sky in a posture typical probably of
every white person who entered, who, like me, was unused to such
innovation in the roof and looked forward to the night when the skyhole
would become a luminous bubble of plastic stars.

The hogan was small and chilly and had the stale odor of having
been closed up with the faint smell of bad breath, deodorant and
perfume of recent retreatants. Sr. Hyacinth opened each of the three
bedroom doors and told me I could pick anyone I wanted because I
would have the hogan to myself, except, of course, when there was an
overflow of retreatants, which didn't happen very often and the empty
bedrooms would be filled. I walked from room to room quickly
scanning for some kind of distinction but even the bedspreads were the
same, tan with ribbing on top. The rooms were very tiny and I could
touch the roof if I wanted, giving the impression I had entered a hobbit
hole. And due to the octagonal shape, hogans are built irregularly
making the structure unique in itself and I half expected to run into
Frodo around every corner.

The room on the left had a view that looked directly into the next
hogan and unless I wanted someone watching me undress I would have
to keep the curtains drawn; the room on the right faced east and would
catch the direct rays of the sun and would be too hot; but the middle
room was just right, having a view that looked down on the city of
Gallup with a background of mountains stretching out far behind the
town.

"I'll take this one," I said, satisfied I had chosen the best overall fit to my spectator nature. Privacy and a moderate temperature; I'll test the bed tonight.

"Right," said Sr. Hyacinth, plunking my suitcase on the end of the bed. And opening the closet door pointed out the closet had two drawers at the bottom. Plenty of space for me, I thought with certainty, about the same as I had in the monastery. And pulling down an attached drop-leaf piece of plywood from the side of the closet, she turned the wooden chair to face it, and said, "It's not the biggest desk, but it will do."

"Ah, Sr. Hyacinth . . ." my conscience getting the better of me. But turning, we were back under the skyhole in the entranceway.

"Here is the kitchen. Sink and refrigerator really. Retreatants eat in the dining room at scheduled times. You won't have to use this kitchen either. Sr. Celeste cleared some space in the main refrigerator for you and we'll eat in the regular dining room off the kitchen.

"Okay, but I have to tell . . ." I started again, but turning, she was under the skyhole again.

"Another innovation to our hogans, thermostats. And where authentic hogans are sometimes made from mud mixed with brush, we used cement. It doesn't look so bad either, you know, log, cement, log, cement, all the way up. It keeps the heat in. Your thermostat is right here," showing me how to turn it on.

"That's fine," I said, relieved I didn't have to haul wood in for a woodstove for a fire as heat. Now that would be primitive.

I ushered her into one of the empty bedrooms and we sat on the end of the bed. "I really want to tell you something," deciding it will be better to begin my volunteer years by honest means. "I debated whether to tell you this or not," I blurted out, "but it's not fair to you if I don't. A few months ago I was diagnosed with multiple sclerosis. It affected my walking the most but as I you can see I'm back to normal. My doctor said sometimes patients go for long times in between episodes, sometimes even years, so I shouldn't have any problems while I'm here. I thought you should know."

I went on, "I received a hopeful letter from a Franciscan superior telling me about the Retreat Center in New Mexico and she forwarded the address of a place they had recently agreed to operate with members of their order. The one line in the letter which stuck in my mind like a challenge was, "Just remember, the Sisters stationed in Gallup have pioneering spirits." It was all the pitch I needed.

Remembering my actions, I told her that's when I wrote to her, as the director of the center, to ask if she could use the extra help of a volunteer. But I was remiss in mentioning I had recently been diagnosed with multiple sclerosis, I confessed, because I didn't want to give any reason to say no. I just hoped retreat work wouldn't be too stressful and would be something I could handle. And even though I wasn't back to my full strength yet, I thought volunteering would be the perfect solution.

Sr. Hyacinth had written back in no time, "If you'd like to be a volunteer here we will welcome the help, so long as you realize the diocese of Gallup is the poorest in all the United States and we won't be able to pay you other than room and board." Considering a couple of months before I was struggling to walk, money was the last thing on my mind. What I was looking for was a monastic-like peace and quiet, a place where I could be attentive to my inner life and my health. That's all. If I could help out, that would be better yet.

"I'm glad you told me," she said with a serious look, no longer sprinkling her comments with laughter. "While you're here, work as long as you want but be sure you get plenty of rest. Don't overdo and you'll be fine. It so happens Sr. Celeste is a nurse. You'll be fine," she said again in such a positive tone I wanted to cry. And swallowing the lump in my throat, I hoped she was right.

"Okay then, if there's nothing else, I'll let you unpack and get settled in, then come over to the kitchen for some dinner. I think there's some left over pizza," she said, her eyes widening in anticipation.

I stood up. "Great!" I let out. And with a sigh of relief, I felt like a ton of worry had been lifted from my shoulders, and I knew I had done the right thing by telling her. God only knows what I would have done if she hadn't been so courageous, learning the fastest way possible that Sr. Hyacinth had the heart of a lion.

Alone in the hogan I sat on my bed and just "felt" by assessing my situation through my feelings. My imagination having calmed, I began thinking about my good fortune: Gallup had turned into a beautiful city right before my eyes, the retreat was more beautiful than I could have imagined, and I was accepted as a retreat worker even with my condition. 'How lucky could I get'? I wondered as I stood up to unpack, hanging my cowboy hat on a hook on the back of the door.

After my few belongings were put away in drawers or hanging in the closet, I walked to the entry and pulled the front door of the hogan closed behind me. I stepped into the fresh air of the yard. and took a cleansing breath of trouble free air, absolved from my worries, breathing freely for the first time today. And grabbing a tall weed growing next to the door, I pulled it out ending its bid of reaching the little sign that read "Brother Sun." "Not on my watch, you don't," I ordered out loud, hoping the rest of the weeds would shrivel up from the tone in my voice. It was a start, but with the promise of pizza waiting for me in the retreat kitchen, I didn't worry about getting the roots.

I tramped back through the course of weeds to the kitchen, and knocked on the door. From inside Hyacinth told me to come in and I found her sitting in a smaller dining room off the kitchen, a platter of pizza welcomed me. Two empty plates were set beside it.

"Here, you better sit down," she said somberly, pushing out my chair. "I'm afraid I have some bad news," as a lightless shade passed over her face. "I just had a phone call. My brother died and I have to go to Tucson," she managed to say as she slowly put one of the plates away. "I'll be gone at least a week."

Chapter 4—Sightseeing

I have done some daft things in my life but deciding to go sightseeing without telling anyone where I was going ranks near the top. Even if I wanted to tell someone, there wasn't anyone around to inform anyway so before I began working on the yard in earnest, I thought this would be the perfect time to go on a relaxing trip sightseeing; no retreats in progress, nothing was pressing, and with Sr. Hyacinth staying an indefinite length of time in Tucson, what she didn't know wouldn't hurt her. Plus, I really wanted to see what was over the next hill.

Besides being a way of seeing interesting sights, sightseeing can also be a delightful way of opening one's inner eye that will forgo the struggle of meditation. A rhythmic stride helps slow the incessant barrage of words to make room for personal insight. I enjoyed wandering alone for this reason, it was a way of reaching my inner spirit with little personal effort. Also, after all the time I spent sitting on the train it would be good to feel my calf muscles ache, and have my side hurt from walking too far, too fast. I looked forward to feeling a shortness of breath in my lungs because of the high altitude and a burn on my face from the sun. I'd welcome dry and chapped lips as a reminder of how frail the body actually was.

So bright and early the next day with the morning light filtering down on the white flowers of chickweed growing in profusion around my hogan, I headed toward the hill in back of the Retreat Center. With the familiar words of Confucius to inspire me, *"a journey of a thousand miles begins with a single step,"* I started out.

Walking to the edge of the hill I stopped to look at the billowy clouds in a background of deepest blue. A feeling of reverence invaded my being as I looked over this physical peace of hills, clouds and endless sky. Quietly I presented myself to the land, introducing my spirit to the energy of the countryside I would be walking through. With a calm mental attitude I acknowledged the beauty of the land and apologized beforehand for any branches I happen to break or grass I would crush, blending the present with the future in a mystical way. I wanted to start my walk feeling calm, centered, and as still as a hidden lake. It was important for me to have my inner spirit be able to reflect the peacefulness of the natural beauty around me.

The clumpy soft ground made for comfortable walking on a terrain dotted with rocks and scattered with bushes and plants having no value other than ground cover, some alive and green, but all outnumbered by a dry withered majority of weeds. Walking through the tumult of weeds I thought how this would be a good place for snakes to hide, and looked down at what was protecting my feet, old garden boots. They protected against snakes in the monastery and they would have to work now. These hard restrictive garden boots were high enough to keep snakes from striking my ankles all right, but there was no comparing them for comfort to the pair of moosehide moccasins I saw an Indian wearing in town that looked pliable enough to let toes wiggle. Mine didn't. At least my boots didn't have snaps, clasps, or fasteners like some boots if I wanted to walk undetected.

It felt good to be able to rely on my own balance so soon after my stay in the hospital so I didn't use a walking stick. I found using one to be more of a hindrance than a help. Now when I walked, my appreciation of natural beauty was avoidably intertwined to a genuine gratitude for my continued good health. For this reason, I feel my spirituality really began after I became sick.

I listened as the fluttering wings of a dove flew off the ground in front of me before continuing my hike.

Perhaps the best thing about sightseeing is never knowing what you will experience: the striking call of a black-throated warbler, the eye-catching turquoise hue of a spring, a pointed artifact off an arrow from a earlier age. More than once I've done a double-take at what I've found or what has found me…

Up ahead, in a rustle of weeds, something caught my attention. As a woman walking alone, I am always on the alert to avoid mishap and misadventure, so before continuing I needed to find out what caused the rustling. The most logical explanation was it probably was a snake. It was the word *probably* that bothered me and until I knew for sure, I didn't feel safe. Creeping up to the spot, I peered through a shrub without being detected. I could see the white tips of two fuzzy ears protruding through an outgrowth of twigs and stems. And to my surprise, attached to the ears was the cutest tawny colored kitten I had ever seen looking confused, lost and alone! What was a kitten doing way out here? It must have been separated from the rest of its litter. What was it living on? Field mice? Lizards?

Being partial to kittens (especially one as cute as this with its prominent ears and short little tail), I had the brilliant idea of taking it back with me to live in my hogan, and for the next half hour we must have looked like a Laurel and Hardy comedy routine with me trying to capture it with awkward grabs with no luck. Clearly it did not want to be caught as I lunged at it over bushes, sidestepped assorted cacti, and followed it through low chaparral. With its little body almost a perfect blend camouflaging its darting in and out of the patches of brown scrub, I couldn't keep up with the blur. Kneeling down, jumping up, trying to head the skittish creature off at every turn was no use, the compact flurry of pent up energy was frightened to death and running for the first of its nine lives.

Grabbing an opportunity of calm, I cautiously advanced toward it until it was almost within my reach, when all of a sudden, a flash of insight ran through me. I don't have many of what I would call insightful flashes, but this one hit me like a ton of bricks and stopped me dead in my tracks. This was not a regular house cat, a *Felis cactus* or even a *F. domesticus*, this was a bobcat! And where an offspring was roaming, the watchful eyes of a full-grown parent was sure to be. I could feel its eyes staring at me from a hiding spot watching me this very second, and immediately I felt all the blood drain from my face as I froze in my tracks.

At that moment, two things about cats came back to me; they have a special organ in the roof of their mouth called Jacobson's organ that allows them to taste what they smell, and if that were true, if a full grown cat had had a whiff of me, would my salty skin make it seem like I was basting in my own juice?

And the second bit of cat trivia I remembered didn't make me feel any better; lying in wait, creeping up, and pouncing, cats were ambush hunters. These images came to me, not one at a time, but in an animated short; alive, attacking and ferocious.

Afraid to move, ever so slowly I straightened up taking one or two fast looks around the locale, hoping against hope my vision wouldn't land on anything that was licking its chops.

Steady does it, I thought, backing away. Don't make any sudden movements. Not knowing what would be considered aggressive posturing to a bobcat, I continued my slow retreat in a non-assertive backward slouch. Then putting one foot up against the side of the other, I was able to advance unhurriedly by turning around to face the other direction. After several yards of walking I broke into a loose trot. With my heart fluttering with dread, I proceeded with a high speed acceleration, one I didn't think even a puma could match.

Moving from this safe spot, I once again set out on course. I started wondering if one of Confucius's seven paths to Nirvana dealt with overcoming fear, either known as from a wild animal, or fear of the unknown. Thinking about the wild feline I was conscious of the fact that I felt the most fear and apprehension when I thought of what *could* have happened if the mother cat had returned. I realized how lucky it was I hadn't put on perfume that morning, my deodorant was strong enough of a dead give away.

I was able to breathe easier when I finally saw the retreat buildings in the distance but when I was close enough to see my hogan on the side of the hill I knew I had made it back safely and let my jangled nerves loosen up after my relaxing day of sightseeing. I happily began kicking my way through the thinning weeds. With a wave of relief I was glad to be in familiar surroundings and allowed myself to laugh at the day's events.

Almost home and exhilarated to have cheated death, I found myself walking faster while I thought about my averted close call and what *could* have happened. With 'how stupid could I have been?' resounding in each of my steps I pulled up and stopped. Looking back in the direction of the bobcat, I realized this was one time I was glad my journey that seemed like a thousand years was almost over.

Chapter 5—Nipping It in the Bud

Maybe the sight of a carpet-like lawn in front of the retreat house would be expecting too much, but I would try to at least have it look like I tried to run a carpet-sweeper over it by the time Sr. Hyacinth returned. A yard sporting a tidied appearance might cheer her, so I made plans for the week she would be gone to trim the unruly growth off the shrubs, collect the dead leaves, and hose down the moss of cobwebs dangling from the long porch. That would wash away the dirt and the look of neglect at the same time.

With my work cut out before me, I picked up the hook and blade pruner and began clipping the branches sticking out bent, bowed and arched on the large juniper shrub directly in front.

The last minute instructions Sr. Hyacinth had given me were of the common sense variety: "If you hear the phone ringing while you're out working, answer with 'St. Francis Retreat' and be sure to write the messages down. You'll need keys. Here's one for the front door and one to the kitchen. Come in when you get hungry. There's enough food in the refrigerator to feed a small army but Sr. Celeste insists on bringing you more in a couple days, just in case, and she'll be able to check on you. Here's her number if you have any problems. What's she like? Oh, you'll like her. She's the one who hung the sign in the kitchen 'God Bless the Cook.' She's French and speaks with an accent so English is her second language but I don't even notice it anymore.

"She's coming to check on me?" I asked, glad for the backup, feeling a little antsy at the thought of being left here by myself. God bless the cook is right, I thought.

"Celeste, you understand, runs our home for girls who have problems, disciplinary, educational or are just plain incorrigible. Many of the girls were placed with us because of violent parents or alcoholic parents or both. Most come from broken homes. You'll meet them when Celeste comes up with the food. Celeste is responsible for them and never goes anywhere without them, if Celeste is home, the girls are home; if Celeste goes out, the girls go out with her. Basically they are good girls that have grown up in unusual circumstances. Take Jessica for instance. By the time she was twelve she had been stabbed in the back by her uncle, literally. And oh, by the way, everybody is everybody's uncle out here."

When Sr. Hyacinth ended her last minute instructions, I helped load her suitcase in the trunk of the car. I told her how sorry I was about her losing her brother, then watched as she backed the white sedan around and went down the drive leaving me alone in the weeds. Yelling one last bit of encouragement at me I heard, "Don't worry, you'll be fiiiiiine," her voice shrinking away with the downhill grade.

I paused to let a flurry of dust settle on the road while I followed the car with my eyes. With the sound of the car growing fainter and fainter, the noise from the engine finally gave way to a noiseless hush and I had to marvel at the quickening quiet. And it was quiet all right, a little too quiet. Looking around at all the hogans filled with empty bedrooms, the vacancies worked to magnify my aloneness and suddenly I felt very vulnerable. Standing in the yard with the silence pressing on my ears, I thought I heard a voice, a whisper at first, but growing in intensity until I could make out what the inaudible shriek inside my head was saying: *get me out of here*!

If I didn't want my imagination to turn into full-blown paranoia, I knew I had to keep my mind off my isolated predicament here in Indianland. The best thing to do would be to throw myself into the yard work and force myself to think of other things. As soon as I started though, images of Indians hiding behind trees or creeping around bushes would sneak into my thoughts. Where was John Wayne when I needed him? I laughed, aware I was trying to trick myself by acting like I wasn't nervous being here by myself. I couldn't picture the Duke doing yard work anyway.

I looked down at my old and scuffed work boots that cleaning and saddle soap hadn't helped; misshapen and warped they definitely weren't Cinderella's slippers. I remembered these broken-in boots were the very boots I wore while gardening during a two year novitiate in a monastery and in an instant I was back in Arizona with the sun beating on my back as I weeded a bean patch…

Anyone who has ever looked at a centipede up close, knows its body is divided into well-marked rings, up to more than a hundred. Looking more closely, the head is covered by a flat shield and has a pair of antennae that are connected with twelve to more than a hundred joints. Strong-toothed mandibles, with under jaws and palps can be seen in the middle that end in a sharp claw, where the poison gland opens. The legs in other segments have spurs and claws and are generally clawed. "All legs, feelers and jaws," is a good way to describe them.

I don't know if this is what Sister was picturing the moment something ran up her pant leg, but in the Arizona desert it could have been anything. In a split second she had to judge its velocity and the effortlessness with which it scrambled up her leg to decide what it was, but from the sheer number of the fast moving centipedes we saw there, it was a safe bet that's what it was.

I was working in the opposite end of the large garden when the yelling broke out. "Something's on me, something's on me!"

It was difficult to jump up from my kneeling position and I was too far away to help but it wouldn't have mattered anyway because she did the only thing she could have done; down went the jeans and immediately I heard a commanding shout of total shock announcing, *"There it is!"* as she pointed at the offending reddish-brown critter as though she had found a criminal. Back up went the denim, and the several hard thuds of a shovel told me its life had been ended. She acted out of shock then fear, I don't think I could have responded as quickly.

Everything went back to normal after the ten seconds of bedlam, now that the dead centipede had been scooped over the garden fence with a shovel. If the Sister harbored any enmity towards the entire class of Chilipoda after that it didn't show, she was right back in the middle of the rows of young asparagus shoots; I located the next stringy pods to pick, repositioned my kneeling pad, and peace once again descended on the monastery's garden.

Looking at the piles of dead weeds in the retreat yard, I knew I was making headway. I was relieved to know I had not seen anything resembling a centipede since getting off the train in Gallup. Maybe the climate was different here but we also did not have a vegetable garden to attract bugs, insects or cooties. I was especially grateful I hadn't seen any in the vicinity of my hogan.

Memories turned up in the retreat yard like an overturned field with the loss of my vocation making me feel about as dead inside as the pile. I thought of all I had lost during the past month, my vocation, my friends, and my health engulfing me in a painful wave of self-pity. Everything was gone and I was alone up here on this hill. I literally had to force myself to 'do what I was doing' as the working monastic axiom prescribed. So I cut, trimmed, and raked and it was working to keep my mind off my losses. I forced myself to think of all I *did* have. With the yard work acting to keep my mind off my troubles, I knew I was making headway.

As I hoed my way along the edge of the walk I admired the shrubs of junipers the walkways wound around. I wondered if the sharp-pointed, needle-like leaves were enough to keep predators away from the red berries or was the pungent oil enough to repel insects. I looked at my boots. And there resting comfortably on my toe was a miller, its dusty wings pulled back like it had taken root. Sorry to bring its piggybacking to an end, I kicked at the air and watched it fly off in a nervous twitter darting abruptly this way and that. One insect is nothing, I thought, as I was swept back to Arizona by another unexpected memory…

It was almost as though I could hear the fast hum of the flying insects round my ears as they ricocheted off me and each other. As the memory invaded my thoughts, I relived the time in the monastery a plague of insects flew in from Mexico and landed on anything green, covering every vegetable in the garden. One minute everything was fine and the next minute there wasn't one green leaf that didn't have a bug gnawing on it.

There was no time to think. The other Sister and I pulled off our scarves; I ran toward the strawberries and the other Sister just errantly ran about, whipping the scarves wildly at the flying insects. But it was no good, there were thousands; if I shooed away twenty, fifty lighted on the same spot. The food we raised for the monastery to live on was being devoured. All our large green leafy plants were infested with the horrid brown insects.

Although they weren't locusts, I thought how we had been hit by a minuscule biblical plague, being in the monastery. In no time at all, less than 30 minutes, we knew we were fighting a losing battle and stopped swatting the veils at them. Wave after wave of the long thin brown bugs flew in and landed, sometimes leap-frogging over the others, dissatisfied with their place in line, doubling and tripling over each other on one leaf, wanting more of the flat vascular structure of the green.

But as fast as they descended, they flew away, leaving our plants stripped down to sickly stubs. It was disheartening to look across the entire garden and see nothing remaining but stick-like nubs where once healthy green leaves had been. If I hadn't seen it with my own eyes, I wouldn't have believed it. I remembered thinking maybe there *was* something to this fasting after all, especially since I usually erred in the opposite direction. It is hard to put into words what I was feeling as I looked over the total devastation of our garden at that moment.

With no one with me at the Retreat to offer help if I had trouble, I told myself to be extra careful. Sure, I could always phone Sr. Celeste in Gallup but taking into account travel time, there was the possibility she would arrive just in time to call for a coroner. I'd have to be extra careful. And as I was combining the piles of weeds into one large pile, I remembered to watch out for snakes, saying to myself, "beware of the molters," repeating another seemingly useless bit of information I picked up in the monastery. I never thought the precautionary advice would ever come in handy outside the monastery, but here it was. Molters, I had learned, are the most dangerous kinds of snakes because they strike out at what they can't see. I started stepping higher over the piles of weeds.

But if it is impossible to see a snake camouflaged in a confusion of weeds, how much harder would it be to check if it's shedding? Snakes usually found me first even if they were blind, remembering how a skinny little snake had slithered straight over the top of the laces of these very boots. How can you avoid what you can't see? The last thing I wanted to do was greet Sr. Hyacinth with an exciting tale of a near miss with a snake.

I put down the shears to ease my aching shoulders and grabbed a shovel which let me use a different set of muscles. I began to hack at a partially exposed root that was feeding an unruly plant on the footpath. It was a useless, thick taproot replenishing an odd plant. Bending in closer, I opened my eyes wider. I could see it was responsible for conducting water, minerals, and food to the out of proportioned, rangy plant, and it was holding the yard back from looking perfect. Aiming the shovel, I came down hard on the ground part. It took three tries to detach it.

In cutting the root, I realized it was not the only thing I severed. Just as the root is an anchor for the plant, I was holding onto memories of my monasticism like a ground; vivid, living memories which in themselves were good-adventurous, dangerous, heartfelt, spiritual, humorous, but now each memory acted like an open wound. Every time I brought one to mind, the sadness at losing a part of my life forever opened.[1] It was an excruciating pain that cut deeply. I kept telling myself "time heals all wounds," so why did it feel like mine were still bleeding?

Taking it out on the root helped. With every hard, energetic hit some of the pain was replaced with a feeling of accomplishment at separating the root from its food source, at doing a service that was sorely needed, at benefiting a bereaved person. I substituted a little at a time but every little bit helped.

Now every hack I took I aimed at memories from the monastery, good and bad, of insects, snakes, and plagues. If I didn't let go of the past, I couldn't fully live in the present. In cutting the root, I was disconnecting sadness at what I had lost. It wasn't until I understood memories, like people, didn't die, they live on in us. In different degrees, I had wrestled with some of the same issues concerning loss this week as Sr. Hyacinth. Nearly finished, I raked up the leftover cuttings and leaves and looked back over the yard complimenting myself on a job well done. I hoped Hyacinth had given her sorrow words like I had this week too.

I had filled one bag after another, laying one on top of another to form a good-sized heap. Grouped together, in one way or another I had lopped off pieces of denial, anger, bargaining, depression, and acceptance, the five stages of grief.[2] Like the yard, I would have to gather the pieces of my hurt again and again until the time came and I reached the point I could easily pass through a day without an expression of pain.

Armed with a new sense of purpose, branches and leaves began flying off the shrubs in furious succession. I applied this renewed vigor on the final pruning until a manicured orderliness was in place. Opening the clippers I went after the last branch sticking out obliquely from the rest, squeezing the handles of the clippers together for the last hard cut. When the sturdy branch fell to the ground in a deadened crack the branch's red berries landed on my boots like drops of blood, it felt like I had cut through a heartstring as well.

As the sun sank deeper over our hill, I began gathering the tools. Soon dusk would settle on the yard in a fine haze. That's when the stout-hearted words of Sr. Hyacinth came back to me, "You'll be fine," she had emboldened. Now that I had finished my inner work, I did feel fine.

Chapter 6—Trailblazers

Ruby! Come back here," a woman's voice scolded when she was turning off the truck's engine. "You know better than to open the door when the car is still moving!"

Looking up, the little girl headed straight for me like a canon ball, totally ignoring the voice from the car.

Coming close she asked bluntly, "Who are you?"

"Anne," I said back to her.

"What are you doing here?" the girl spoke out again without a hint of inhibition.

"Picking up the yard," making my answers as short as her questions.

"What for?" she burst out, unable to understand why a stranger would be cleaning the yard of the Retreat Center.

"Don't you think it needs it?" I said, nodding my head in the direction of the weeds near the hogans and the overgrowth on the walkways.

"I guess you're right," the dark-haired little girl approved, happy to have made conversation before she would be told to stop bothering me.

"What's your name?" it was my turn to ask.

"Ruby. I live at Sr. Celeste's house, Our Lady of Perpetual Help Home for girls," she said proudly, honored to have been selected to live at the private school. "Good for you," I said.

Together with her pluckiness, I noticed there was something different about her looks which was hard to pinpoint, not deformed, just different, and somehow it fit with her forward demeanor. Her small dark eyes were slightly crossed and she had a wide upturned nose and thin lips. Excluding her Navajo accent, she still would have been hard to understand. Unclear in communicating her thoughts, she easily reached her frustration level and shouted, "I'm not doing anything wrong," at the Sister closing in from behind, the girl's impulsive behavior annoying the guardian in the on-going struggle.

The other girls soon caught up to Ruby. "They live with me and Sister."

"Hi," an older girl spoke up, eating something out of a white paper bag. In between swallows she said, "I'm Joyce. And this is Valerie, Daniel, Molly, Virginia, and Jessica," motioning to each successively. "We all live with Ruby."

"I'm Anne, a volunteer."

Joyce, a teenager wearing jeans and plaid shirt, kept fingering something in the small white bag. Noticing her fidgeting, to break the ice I asked, "Donuts?" just to make conversation.

"No, they're chilies. Want one?"

The question was asked innocently enough. What harm could there be in tasting one? Besides, I didn't want to look like a lightweight at our very first meeting. I enjoy spicy food and I like hot salsa, and after all, this kid was nibbling on one. "How hot could they be? If she could do it, I certainly could." Was I wrong! I couldn't keep it in my mouth! Immediately it erupted into angry snaps all over my mouth, lips, gums, tongue, each seed igniting a fire of its own, to the friendly delight of the watching Navajo girls now doubled over with laughter.

"Water!" I said, fanning my mouth.

"Hello," I heard from the approaching footsteps walking up from the truck. "I'm Sr. Celeste," the heavily accented voice directed. "I came up to see if you needed anything."

"Water!" I repeated, really playing it up so the girls would get the most mileage they could out of their practical joke.

"Here drink this," Sister encouraged, handing me a can of soda.

"Thanks," I choked out turning toward the voice. Through watering eyes I could make out a Sister in a black habit and veil like Hyacinth's, only a size smaller. Other than the heels Celeste had on her black pumps, she looked like a miniature Hyacinth.

"I tried to catch you before they did. The trick is not to chew, but even so, chilies are hot."

"Yes, they are! I've never tasted anything so hot!" which brought on another burst of laughter from the girls. It was beyond me how something so hot could taste good to them, but then again, maybe they didn't have any tastebuds left. Drawing a cool breath in and out through my mouth with a *whoosh*. I did so over and over.

"I see you've met the girls." She turned to them and in her beautiful French accent Sr. Celeste introduced Valerie, Daniel, Molly, Virginia, and Jessica. And of course, Ruby. Voila. These are my girls."

"*Yah-te-hey*," they responded in unison with the Navajo greeting for hello, each girl giving me a shy smile as her name was called.

Apologizing for Ruby's pushy behavior, Sr. Celeste announced "She's a fetal alcohol syndrome baby."[3] This caused Ruby to grin from ear to ear as if she had been had been awarded a prize.

Without the hint of self-consciousness, Ruby visibly swelled when her special contribution to the home was declared. "I turned sixteen this week," announcing this benchmark in her life with pride.

"Wow," I said, making my surprise at how young she looked act like merry-making. She actually looked about thirteen.

"Girls, this is Anne." Sr. Celeste broke in, ending Ruby's responses. "She is a volunteer and helping Sr. Hyacinth at the Retreat."

Deciding beforehand I wouldn't say anything about my being at a monastery and risk looking like a prude. And I wouldn't say anything about having multiple sclerosis either and risk looking like a weakling. I simply said, "I'm Anne and I'm from Los Angeles."

"A volunteer?" all the girls spoke in unison, "You're working here for free?" bewildered why anyone from anywhere would want to work without getting something in return.

"You mean like Fred was?" Valerie, one of the older girls asked.

"Yes, but ladies volunteer too, pointing the girls in the direction of the truck to help her unload the food she had prepared.

"Who is Fred?" I asked Sr. Celeste as we all walked to the truck. And as if the train had been cued, the loud smooth whistle blasted in the distance effectively ending the subject and my question about Fred was hustled aside by Sister. In a murmured sigh from her, I heard "poor Fred," under her breath and dropped the subject.

"Girls, please help me unload the food from the truck. Everyone grab something and take it into the kitchen. There is a retreat this weekend."

"A retreat? This weekend?" I asked in an anxious voice. Suddenly poor Fred didn't seem so important anymore. Compared to this, nothing did because I would find out if I was suited to a retreat vocation or not.

"You mean Hy didn't tell you? Sometimes she can be so forgetful. Isn't that just like Hyacinth?"

"I don't know. Is it?" All I knew about her was what I learned on the ride from the train station, now more grateful than ever she remembered to pick me up.

"Sometimes Sr. Hyacinth has a short memory, it's true," Sr. Celeste said, "but I can understand why with her brother's death and all. Come on, we better check on what the girls are up to," leading the way to the retreat kitchen. "Sometimes they get into the desserts."

We found the girls sitting quietly in the small dining room each with a glass of chocolate milk in front of them. "They said it was all right," Ruby was first to explain, unaware of the mustache of chocolate on her upper lip. "They told me to," pointing at the others.

"It's okay," Celeste said wiping at Ruby's mouth. "Go outside and run off the sugar. You know what it does to you Ruby."

Rinsing their glasses and leaving them by the dishwasher like it was their normal routine while visiting, they politely walked out the door and into the yard to play.

I think I'm going to like the Navajo culture, I thought, if all of them are as polite and courteous as these girls. The impression I had was they were bright and intelligent (they already knew two languages, at least), they had been friendly and curious in wanting to know who I was and where I was from and what I was doing here. And even if I was the object of some good good-natured teasing, I appreciated their sense of humor. Stemming from their calm demeanor was a quiet reserve; natural, unhurried, and content. I couldn't help admiring a community that turned out such contented people, people who know who they are, that feel so at home. Somehow it made me want to be a better person. I caught myself standing straighter.

"Come sit down Anne," Sr. Celeste said. "We'll have our own cup of chocolate."

I sat at the table off the kitchen across from Celeste looking at the view through the sliding glass doors. We were high on the retreat hill and the fields were shimmering flaxen in the afternoon sun and I told her, "the view beats staring at the back of a cereal box any morning," watching her pour our milks.

"Ruby is an alcohol syndrome baby," she began. "I'm sure you've noticed some differences physically. She has developmental problems too. She can be difficult at times but on the whole she's just a trusting little girl. She has problems with her attention and explodes at the slightest provocation. I wanted you to be aware of this. Both her mother and father were alcoholics and that can have disastrous effects on a fetus. Alcohol can have bad effects on all pregnant women, Navajo or not." Watching Celeste drink, I remembered Sr. Hyacinth told me Celeste was a nurse.

"It's never too early for the girls to start learning about the effects of alcohol. About all I can do," she said, "is tell the girls how easily alcohol crosses the placenta and that burying parts of the afterbirth has nothing to do with preventing birth defects. But trying to change life rituals is a struggle as difficult as changing eating habits; like substituting vegetables for *fry bread*, a favorite food. But nothing works better than the example of Ruby, and making sure they know Ruby's condition was absolutely preventable. To inflict this kind of suffering on a child is unthinkable.

"Gallup," she reminded, "has programs to educate women of the risks of drinking during pregnancy, but many still believe in the old world ways; burying the umbilical cord near the family home will transfer support from the biological mother to Mother Earth and burying the placenta near a young tree will help nourish an infant so both will grow strong."

"That's so interesting," I said, taken out of my customary way of thinking. "I love learning about Indian culture."

"It will surprise you how much you'll learn when you're here," Sister said, nodding her head.

"The 'Blessing Way' ceremony is another version I know where the placenta is buried in a cornfield to tie the child to the land. It's also used for protecting sheep herds and warriors, and not just expectant mothers."

"There are all kinds of interesting cultural differences. For instance, have you ever heard of a cradleboard? I'll show you one when we're in town sometime. It's a wooden bed made from cottonwood, pine or cedar laced together with strips of leather, like a portable papoose. Navajos believe its flat boards will give a baby a straight back. And the supporting pad will give the baby a nice rounded head. It's cut from the same tree where the placenta is buried. The spiritual relationship between the child and the tree lasts the life of a child.

"Sr. Hyacinth and I went through our own learning process. We found out soon enough after we opened the home how a hurtful past can lead to problems in behavior," Celeste said with a serious face. "We learned how important it is to have every cruel and hurtful incident in childhood be told to someone other than a relative or friend, someone trained to handle all kinds of trauma so we hired a counselor. I think I can speak for Hyacinth in saying hurt sometimes speaks louder than the heart."

We moved into the kitchen and could hear playful shouts coming from the yard as we rinsed out our glasses. Looking out the window overlooking the yard towards the yells, it wasn't long before we had been spotted. With the steady sound of footsteps approaching, in walked a flushed face Ruby who immediately threw her arms around Sr. Celeste's neck and demanded, "I want to go home," brusquely.

"In a minute. Can't you see Anne and I are talking?" she reminded, as she tried to pry Ruby's arms from her neck. Unable to extricate herself from Ruby's iron grip, Celeste finally said, "It would take more than a medicine man to chant the wayward spirit out of Ruby."

Standing at the top of the drive waving good-bye, I could see Ruby waving frantically at me from the back seat as they pulled away. I remembered Sister's last remark, but thought if anyone needed the healing power of the Blessing Way chant to release a wayward *anything*, it wasn't Ruby, it was her parents.

Images of chilies, cradleboards, and medicine men passed through my mind while I followed the sound of their car on the ribbed road to the paved highway. But as fascinating as my mental pictures were, right now nothing was more important to me than remembering we were having a retreat this weekend. This was *the* weekend, the one everything boiled down into; the train ride, the Sisters, the hogans. This was the weekend I would find out if I had a retreat vocation or not. And if I didn't, with no job, little money and ill-health, what would I do?

I had a lot riding on this weekend.

Chapter 7—Tall Spirits

At first when I saw the figure standing rigidly erect in the back of the pickup following Sr. Hyacinth's car, I thought she brought back her dead brother with her. And by the way she was shouting loud commands at the truck driver, "Too far left! Too far right!" to keep him from veering off the driveway and onto the walkways. Escorting him around the tree in front, I knew she had postponed her mourning period indefinitely until after the work was done. She was doing what made her feel better, taking charge, and she was good at it too. A solemn funeral procession it wasn't.

"Look what my brother left the retreat!" Sr. Hyacinth yelled happily, as she climbed out of her car. Pointing, she directed my attention to the cargo in the back of the truck like I may have missed it.

"Just look at it!" she called out again.

I walked to the back of the truck and the driver opened the tail gate to give us an unobstructed view of the tall figure. All three of us stood there momentarily sizing up the molded likeness.

"Jesus!" I said, my eyes widening. "It certainly is big." No mistaking it, this larger than life statue was definitely a replica of Jesus. Its stiff figure had been wrapped in a furniture pad for the transit, all but the arms, they were sticking straight out from its sides in the form of a T, built-in perches for birds. But because I only knew Sr. Hyacinth a few days at this point, I was relieved to see it wasn't a large ceramic wood nymph.

As the driver pulled the furniture pad from the statue, Sr. Hyacinth beamed, "Isn't it a good likeness?" tugging at a corner of the heavy pad to hurry the momentous unveiling. "My brother was going to donate it to the retreat, his wife told me. Too bad he won't get to see it here. He would be happy to know it finally made it."

Anxious to hear what I thought of the lily white Jesus, she asked me again, "Tell me, don't you think it's a wonderful likeness?"

Now I didn't know that much about the craft of statuary art but I thought this figure of Jesus was a good one. Tasteful and simple in its porcelain-like purity. In this unpainted state it was so white, so white in fact, it looked like it was giving off an aura. "I like it," I said, meaning it. "It will have a lively effect on the yard," making a mental note to poke my head out hogan door tonight to see if it glowed in the dark.

"I thought we'd put it right over here," walking quickly to the spot in front. "That way people will make no mistake they were entering a Catholic retreat center. What do you think?"

I agreed. "I think that is just the right place," looking at the open arms of Jesus like they were wings. "It does give an overall feeling of *welcome*. And you're right, it's so big no one will miss it," glad she would have a visible reminder of her brother every time she stepped into the yard.

Actually I was hoping she would have a sign made while she was gone. We needed a sign, something like St. Francis Retreat. Maybe with an attached donation marker: this sign generously donated by the Beloved Brother of Sister Hyacinth to keep his memory alive.

"It weighs a ton," the driver remarked, "so wherever you decide you'd like me to put it, it stays. One other thing. Sorry but my boys knocked off two fingers from the left hand when they were loading it, but like I was saying, it weighs a ton."

Hoping to avoid a lengthy repair job, Hyacinth asked, "Anne, do you think you could fix it?"

Surprised at myself, I said, "I can't believe I'm saying this, but yes, I think I can," remembering how I worked with plaster of Paris in the monastery making mosaics.

The driver reached in his pocket and took out the two fingers and handed them to me. "One index-finger, and one finger next to it," he said, handing over the responsibility for fixing it to me.

Assured everything was coming together Sr. Hyacinth walked to the spot where she wanted the statue to stand and stretching out her arms said, "Right here."

It was to the left of the driveway, in one of my recently weeded plots. The driver backed the truck up to the place, lowered the tailgate and climbed in. In a penguin walk from side to side, he moved the heavy statue to the very edge of the truck and giving a long strenuous heave, slid the statue to the ground on a furniture mat into its permanent resting place.

"There you go, Sister," he said, slapping his hands together in finality. And asking Hyacinth to sign something, he climbed back into the cab, and hightailed it back to Tucson before Sr. Hyacinth could find anything else for him to do.

Together, Sister and I walked up to the very front of the property so we could get the full impact pretending to be retreatants. Even minus the two fingers, it was an impressive sight standing fast like a lighthouse, arms open wide, beckoning all who pass by with its bold white eloquence. "Well, I like it," she said. "If it could talk he would be big-sounding like my brother. A fine memento to remember my brother by. Don't you think? It really adds to the yard."

I followed Sister as she circled it. After deliberating, while looking at his face, she finally exclaimed, "I know what's missing! He doesn't have any eyes!" Meaning, he didn't have any color in his pupils. I had noticed this too, like rigor mortis had set in making it stare straight ahead. "Anne, as long as you're fixing the fingers, do you think you can add a little color to his eyes to make it look human?"

Pupils are small, I thought, how could I mess up such a small job? and Hyacinth was set on having a bold Jesus eye-balling the Retreat. Plus it would make it look better because right now it had a blank stare. I answered her with, "Sure, I'll give it a try."

It didn't end up like *Christ the Redeemer* in Rio de Janeiro, but it did cordially welcome people. I was pleased.

Poised over the eyes I cautioned myself, the lighter, the better when I painted the eyebrows in so it wouldn't end up looking like Groucho Marx.

I secured the detached fingers with globs of plaster of Paris on each knuckle, scraping the excess away until two perfectly aligned digits were in place, complete with fingernail indentations I outlined with a stick. I only hoped the fingers wouldn't fall off during snow and rain and wash away. A retreatant finding dirty, lifelike fingers washed up in a puddle somewhere would ruin their whole retreat experience.

I had to find the right type of paint for the eyes. Flat, latex, water base, acrylic? Something with a shine might make his eyes look beady, I thought. And I avoided any color that had a hint of red to it that would make his eyes look bloodshot. Black, dark brown, auburn, chestnut and gray, these were the colors I had to choose from out of Retreat's art supply closet.

Aware the tall white figure with its arms extended already looked imposing even if it didn't have a flood light at night, it couldn't be missed in headlights, I painted in the black eyes of a mid-easterner at first but it made it look possessed, so I wiped off what I could and applied the dark brown, then the next color, then the next, going through all the shades I had. But whatever I used as careful as I was, it somehow ended up with the kind of eyes that followed to the left and to the right; wherever I was. It was unnerving, and I hoped it wouldn't scare the retreatants. It would be all right I told myself as long as it was viewed from a distance.

Looking at it, I thought of what St. John of the Cross wrote on the use of images: that "…those who have images so ill-carved that they *take away* devotion rather than produce it, for which reason some image-makers who are very defective and unskilled in this art should be forbidden to practice it." *(Ascent of Mount Carmel*, St. John of the Cross, Book III.) I thought my painting the pupils a muted brownish-black would keep him from turning over in his grave.

A few days later when the repair work on the statue was finished, I brought Sr. Hyacinth out to show her.

"That's fine. And a good job on the fingers, you can't even tell they have been reattached," inspecting my work at close range. "But those eyes. I love what you did with the eyes. They seem to look right through me it was looking into my soul," pleased with the repairs.

"You know what else would be nice?" she asked. "Let's bring one on the little benches from the porch and put it right in front of the statue, that way a retreatant can have a personal meditation here without distractions. "What do you think?"

Smiling at her, I said, "Come on. Let's get it."

And as we walked to the porch together, I could feel a lightness in my step as I recalled the month's occurrences—from the yardwork, advice given in French accents, alcoholic syndrome babies, a traveling Jesus, masonry, and optical illusions, I had learned three important things about retreat work: 1) an important quality for any staff member to have is an accommodating nature 2) with this kind of variety I will never be bored and 3) most importantly, I was going to enjoy retreat work immensely.

When we reached the porch, Hyacinth pulled up suddenly and exclaimed, "By the way, the yard looks great!"

Chapter 8—A World Apart

The thin afternoon air was heavy with the excitement of a housewarming, for Friday was the day most retreats begin, and company was indeed coming. Swirling around the newly sculpted and trimmed look of the yard was a verve and vigor of expectation as I pictured the whole weekend in my head many times; an attractive yard ready for pleasant walks, footpaths cleared like country lanes, an order of peace and tranquillity to help reflect a caring and prayerful atmosphere to assist in the inner journeys of retreatants.

I pictured the dining room filled with the happy sounds of hungry diners looking forward to epicurean delights, women especially feeling like they were in the lap of luxury not having to cook for an entire weekend. And I could see mothers wishful of their favorite food but settling for anything knowing they wouldn't have to sink their hands into dirty dishwater when the meals were over. I visualized men with their mouths watering with unquenchable appetites turning the retreat weekend into an all-you-can-eat marathon, and hoped Sr. Celeste prepared enough food to enable them to go back for seconds if they wanted, making a mental note on their arrival to see who looks like they would take two bites of a cherry pie and put the fork down, and who looked like they could eat two whole cherry pies.

Having seen the guest roster for the weekend consisting of three vegetarians in a total of twenty-seven retreatants, I wondered how Celeste could manage. Did it mean cooking three separate dishes for each special diet for every meal? And how much? Who can predict appetites? I realized then what a stressful job the cook has of planning, ordering, and doing the actual cooking. I knew I wouldn't want it.

I never took the cook's job for granted from then on because I realized the significant contribution they make to retreat work; if the food is terrible, it is a direct reflection on the overall retreat. "What a great weekend!" a retreatant may witness to, when really they're thinking of the boneless braised meat they had the night before. But if the food tastes bad, "That blueberry pie was the worst tasting gruel I ever ate!" it may be used as an excuse when no spiritual insights are forthcoming. If every bite enraptures the retreatant in a blissful out-of-body experience of the palate, they'll leave fulfilled, enlightened from head to toe and give favorable reviews of the entire weekend. Such is the influential power food has over a retreat, the cook serving up a spiritual bill of fare.

I knew our Retreat was the perfect reserve for quiet prayer. It overlooked the city of Gallup and the chapel was built on the side of a hill especially for the impressive view. I remembered how Sr. Hyacinth purposely waited until it was dark before taking me inside so she could show it off, and it worked. I was awestruck. As soon as I walked in I was taken by the twinkling city lights that flooded the large floor-to-ceiling windows. It was like I was looking down on a city of jewels and seeing the New Jerusalem, the final resting place of redeemed souls. Gallup from this angle appeared to be the most ideal community on earth.

"Are you looking for a quiet place so you can find God?" the flyer for this weekend read. But everywhere I looked I was surrounded by wide open spaces, except Gallup's metropolis, so I wondered if this was their best selling point.

Hyacinth told me Gallup's faithful liked the old-fashioned kind of retreats, so St. Francis Retreat catered to the more traditional themes of prayer, supplication and Scripture. "You know, the important things," she explained. "Like the retreat this weekend: 'The Protection of Prayer,' and how we find a defense in God by practicing mercy and compassion toward others. "Not that this should create a false sense of security in life, mind you."

"What do you mean?" I asked, watching her as she was separating the vestments in the closet in the sacristy in the chapel, pulling out the right color vestment for the liturgical season in front.

"To answer your question Anne, you wouldn't deliberately put yourself in harms way, say by taking a walk at midnight down a dark alley in the worst part of town and expect God to ward off all dangers, would you?"

"I should think not," agreeing with her, following her as she moved over and began sorting through the numerous hanging white albs making sure they were clean for the visiting Priest.

"In fact, I heard a question that will help get us into the mind set of this retreat. What do you think God's greatest gift to man is?"

"Ah, well I…"

"That even though he sees famine and disease, death and destruction all around, he never thinks it will happen to him!" she said, almost laughing. "This is God's greatest gift to man."

Waiting momentarily, I answered, "That's so true, but there are exceptions; if people had a chaotic childhood, then they'll wonder when the next disaster is going to strike and be on guard," speaking from experience.

With a wry smile, she looked at me and said, "I guess there's an exception to everything. It's something for us to think about anyway." She pushed the long, white hanging under-garments together, smoothing the white material as flat as they could be, and closed the closet door.

"Okay, we're done here," she said, referring to running through the particulars in the sacristy. Because of the time I spent in the monastery, I understood most of what she was talking about. I just didn't know where things where kept-keys, hosts, incense, matches, monstrance. These were small easy-to-forget items, but missing any one of them could bring a service to a halt. I made a mental note to check and replenish each after every retreat.

"Now I have to get back to the office and finish some paperwork," she stated emphatically. "There's always someone who calls asking for directions. Were running out of time," Sister said.

"Yes, I know. I still have a few things I want to do too," I said, but I was thinking how I wasn't going to let anything disrupt the retreat weekends I had planned in my mind: beautiful grounds ready for strolling, delicious food for body and mind, a reflective place for worship and prayer in the chapel; an entire weekend designed to take the retreatants away from their everyday world. This wouldn't be an average weekend for them. I wanted it to be perfect.

I hadn't planned on retreatants arriving well before the scheduled time destroying my last minute preparations, early morning instead of early evening.

"Hello there, I'm Mrs. Blatt" surprising me with the excuse, "I wanted to get some quiet time in before the rest of the crowd arrived." And while I could see her point, it was a startling surprise, like someone had thrown a gutter ball and all I could do was watch as it rolled slowly down the channel, ending with the inevitable klunk of her suitcase on the ground.

Mrs. Blatt was a large woman wearing a brightly colored flower-print dress. She was constantly looking around and it gave me the impression she was looking for the dining room because of the telling look of hunger in her eyes. What do I do when a retreatant arrives hours early? The Priest facilitator hasn't even arrived yet. But truthfully, because she was my very first retreatant, this contretemps didn't matter much. She didn't know it at the time, but she taught me something I would carry with me from then on as retreat professional; to *expect* retreatants hours before the retreat started as the *norm*.

I greeted her with, "Welcome, I'm Anne. Let's go to the office to see if your room's ready," stalling for time because everything wasn't quite ready. It was when I walked her to the office that I realized in one fell swoop she had destroyed my time schedule for the morning.

I introduced Mrs. Blatt to Hyacinth who signed her in. After Hyacinth gave her a short welcome, the retreatant was given a room key and the brief itinerary for the weekend.

"You may make coffee if you like," was the hospitable thing to offer. I hadn't planned on classifying retreatants on the their ability to adapt to an unfamiliar coffee maker. As it turned out, I should have. I found out it was quite possible for someone using a bigger, unfamiliar coffee maker to forget to use a paper filter and have boiling water squirt from around the rim of the metal holder, sending hot water cascading over the counter flooding the floor. Use of the kitchen was forfeited for a while and I had to post a "kitchen closed" notice on the door to alert Sr. Celeste who would be coming at any time to start dinner, bringing the girls up with her. I didn't know what a group going through caffeine withdrawal was capable of but it couldn't be helped. Not to mention the scarcity of sugar from being withheld from the gratis snack food of sweet rolls and other delights all of which were homemade.

As more and more retreatants descended on the Center with their nervous energy, talking and laughing, images of how the retreat should progress ran through my mind. I wasn't about to let a few minor setbacks get in the way of a perfectly good retreat weekend, my very first one. I still pictured guests taking meditative walks, listening intently to the facilitator in the conference room, contemplatively praying in the privacy of the chapel…

"There's a strange odor in my bedroom. It smells like something died," the woman barely choked out.

Now what? I thought, as I shrank back.

"I'm sure you're mistaken," I apologized, while searching the grounds for Hyacinth at the same time, she would know what to do. I followed the middle aged woman to her hogan to assess the situation for myself.

Flinging open the door of the hogan with one hand and covering her nose with the other, I followed her in. "See," she sputtered.

There was no mistaking it. The foul odor was indeed emanating from inside her hogan like decaying flesh, the putrid smell sticking in my throat like a month old ham. I had to move her to another room.

Ushering her out the door in a hurry, I apologized profusely, assuring her the hogan didn't smell like this yesterday but I could tell my expression of regret did little to ease her concerns. Although I wasn't sure if I should, I assigned her to a room in the brand new building because I thought she'd had enough of an authentic hogan for one day.

I walked back into the yard again and steeled myself before entering the smelly hogan to scour the rooms for the source of the odor. It wasn't hard to find the culprit; a dead squirrel, tangled and stiff and stuck in the coiled metal springs underneath one of the beds. "Poor Rocky, what a terrible way to go," I thought, as I carefully extricated its little carcass by using a newspaper left in the closet. I began checking the other rooms to see if he'd brought any friends in with him.

"Out with the bad, in with the good." I breathed, flipping the last mattress over in the foul smelling hogan. I was relieved when I didn't find any more skeletal remains trapped in the springs. One was bad enough. Straightening up, I walked through the hogan opening all the windows to air it out before pulling the door closed behind me.

Hopefully the smell will be gone in a couple of weeks, I thought, still taking deep gulps of fresh air. And what about what jumped off of it while it was trapped in there? Anything from ticks and mites to worms and lice. These diseased laden parasites would have to be dealt with by sterilizing the entire bed, mattress, springs, pad. Would Lysol give any protection from rabies? Walking out in back of the retreat, I placed him in the metal trash and replaced the lid.

My role at the retreat became apparent and came naturally to me. With Sr. Hyacinth busy with the business end of it assigning rooms and taking money, and Sr. Celeste busy preparing meals, I had to see to everything else because with our skeleton staff, there *was* no one else. I felt like a human pinsetter setting things straight and seeing that everything was properly set and in uniform condition. Making sure the retreat got off to a successful delivery became my job and I took it seriously. I loved being a spiritual docent.

I wanted to give retreatants the chance to experience a perfect retreat weekend. 'Perfect' meaning, I wanted to give them every opportunity of feeling the twinges of the mystical by keeping all mundane concerns and disquieting distractions at a minimum so they could concentrate on their inner lives, not on leaky coffee makers or strange smells, for instance. By keeping things running smoothly, I felt I could insulate them from the cares of the world. Then theoretically, a retreatant would be unobstructed enough to receive enlightenment and insights. This was my plan.

I hoped it wasn't noticeable but I could feel agitation rising to my face in flustered feelings at having my morning time schedule destroyed, embarrassment at having to limit the use of the kitchen cutting off refreshments, the horrific discovery of a dead and possibly diseased squirrel. It made me think, "What did that wise man say about disease, death and destruction?" Ruefully I questioned why it had to happen all on the same day.

I had to admit though, I never thought it would happen to me.

Chapter 9—Bedsitter People

Vocations today have gone the way of the world. Chopping wood for fires is replaced with short walks to the thermostat to move the indicator up on easier electric heaters, while self-initiative in individuals has dipped as low as an April temperature in the high desert. One can almost hear the rush to an easier lifestyle in cushioned soles. When everything is handed over in a drawstring bag, it's hard to expect the opposite; and this softness is recognized as laziness. Placing the hand stamped sterling necklace back around their neck, the last line heard on the way out: "It was too hard."

Invaluable contributors are missionary Sisters, whose main concern is to attend by word and deed. Hard-working and selfless, dedicated missionaries go where they are needed feeling obliged by the weight of necessity. "Thus it was, and has always been, the task of missionaries working within the system to bring spiritual hope and physical sustenance to oppressed people, given typically limited authority, resources, and income."[4] Sr. Carol fit into this category like the inlay on her pocket knife. She was of medium height with a wiry build, this plucky nun, seventy-ish, was feisty as the devil and had the habit of giving to Peter what may have belonged to Paul when no one was around, earning her a reputation as being devilishly angelic, depending on who you talked to and where their affiliation lay, with Peter or with Paul. She belonged to a nearby parish that had a church built in the shape of an umbrella, a very large wooden umbrella, and I wondered if everyone who prayed there was inclined to invoke God for good weather like I did. That's where I was introduced to her, after a Sunday Mass and I had a feeling, as a missionary, she would make a good contact.

St. Jerome's Church had two very large floor to ceiling stained glass panels of St. Jerome and Our Lady of Guadalupe greeting all who entered. The first time I walked up the stone steps and pushed opened the heavy wooden doors of the church, my eyes were immediately drawn to a beautiful parallel of color. But casting my sight beyond the windows on the view I saw white tufts of fog hugging the hill below in an endless line of rumpled satin. No glasswork could ever capture such natural beauty. I knew about the Our Lady of Guadalupe. I had the privilege of piecing together Her likeness in a glass mosaic when I was in the monastery in Arizona and came to know every inch of the colorful design intimately and of the miracles she performed for a poor Indian.

I didn't know about St. Jerome until I read a brief summary on a plaque in the back of the church about his life. I felt an immediate kinship with him: "The lion could not speak, since it was not his nature, but came forward and showed Jerome his wounded paw. It was full of thorns, and was swollen and feverish. Jerome called the brothers to come with warm water and clean cloths and healing herbs. Then he pulled out the thorns, while the lion looked gratefully into his face and tried not to howl…When the paw healed, the lion became gentle as a lamb."[5]

I felt drawn to his warm affinity time and time again because I have come to see emotional scars from childhood as invisible thorns that have to be removed before healing takes place. And in the back of my mind, I admit, like the gentleness given to St. Jerome's lion, I wondered if I would be changed somehow when I am finally healed.

On the left side of the church, the same side as the artwork of St. Jerome, was a large gnarled piece of mesquite heavily coated with lacquer. It was covered with dark knots and deep uneven crevices that and stood about six feet tall. The longer I looked at it, the ferocious head of a lion would take shape, obviously the artist's intention. Between the Lady of Guadalupe and St. Jerome, the church embodied some very important phases in my life. So much so, when I pushed open the doors to the church, it felt like I was pushing open doors to my karma and I would bask in this feeling of synchronicity under the watchful eyes of the carved out piece of burl.

I suppose it was curiosity that would make me sit and try to understand this distinctive feeling I had every time I entered St. Jerome's church. It was during one of these ruminative moments while by myself in the church, deep in thought, that I heard a loud honk from a car horn that blasted me back to the present. I walked to the back of the church and opened the door a crack. I could see it was the missionary Sr. Carol sitting behind the wheel of a mud-splattered Ford Bronco. It occurred to me as I was stepping out to talk to her, that in her line of work—visiting the poor and attending the needy—over remote reservation land communities, unlike her city counterparts that only went off-roading when they accidentally backed over a flower bed, she actually needed to drive a four-wheel-drive vehicle. I was about to find out.

"Yah-te-hey! Anne!" she screamed from the driver's side window. "Want to go with me to the reservation?"

I wasn't about to turn down an opportunity to go on the reservation so, knowing my work was done for the day, without hesitating I pulled the church doors closed behind me and yelled back, "Let's go! Just let me tell Sr. Hyacinth where I've gone." Taking the steps two at a time, I ran to the office, and was back climbing up into the passenger seat ready for my first visit to the reservation.

Hanging from the rear view mirror was a circle made out of bark with feathers dangling from two broken arrows intersecting the center, reminding me of a large charm bracelet, not ornamentally, but with beads and string interlaced in meaningful fashion. At the bottom hung a miniature drum and a tiny leather pouch.

"This is a replica of a Medicine Wheel," she said, noticing how taken I was with it. "It's a symbol of peace and tranquillity and is used to ward off evil spirits. I use it to ward off bad drivers."

"Does it work?" I asked, as I noticed there were no seat belts.

"So far," she said, with a smile, adding, "But the peace pipe fell off just last week."

"I hope that isn't an omen," worried it symbolized a tire as the next thing to fall off. I could see myself explaining to an officer about the loose lug nuts, "It was our fault, we did have a sign!"

Sr. Carol pointed at something hanging from her mirror. "These represent the four sacred directions which, when you think of them as a Navajo, are really six: east, west, north, south, and up and down." Made out of little bits of timber, the four sections that were marked by arrows, represent the usual four directions, she told me.

Turning the car around, Sister aimed it downhill into a fog bank. She drove us through to the sunny and bright patches at the bottom of our steep hill that ran alongside the retreat center, and gunning the engine, we took off.

"How far is it?"

And remembering what Sr. Hyacinth told me when I first arrived, I heard the exact line she warned about, "Just down the road a piece."

"What do I have to lose?" I thought. What could happen with a seventy-year-old nun driving?

She pulled us across the main highway leaving the smooth, level, man-made road behind and turned onto the dirt roads of the reservation, full of bumps, holes, and pockets of mud where somebody had emptied something along the way. I noticed how clean the vista was without the usual billboards or signs. I didn't see any hotels or shops for that matter either. There were no road signs whatsoever, we only passed an occasional homestead with hogan, and after about an hour, I asked her, "How do you know where you're going?" trusting in her sense of direction turning this way and that.

"When you've been over these roads as many times as I have, you remember," she said decisively. On the way she told me about her undertakings as teacher, nurse, sympathetic listener. An original good Samaritan, doing whatever was needed.

It was nearly dark when we pulled up in front of Leonard's hogan. Maybe steadying herself by holding on to the steering wheel helped, but these roads didn't phase her in the least; Sr. Carol was as rugged as the Southwest itself.

We drew close to the front of the dark hogan and turned off the engine. Trying to peer into the hogan from the front seat of the Bronco, we could make out what seemed to be someone or something in there, but we couldn't be sure. We could see what looked to be a hunched over figure, dark and motionless, like it had been turned into stone. Cautiously I transferred my weight to my right foot as I slid down from the car, keeping one eye on the vacant door and one eye on Sr. Carol close in front of me.

With much trepidation, we approached the forbidding hogan which seemed as still as a mausoleum. To my surprise as we drew closer, there wasn't a front door to knock on. It was there, but it was off its hinges and placed on its side propped against a rock next to a large barrel out in front. (Hogan doors act like thermostats: off in summer, on in the winter). Without a door, anything or anyone, could have wandered in and the thought made me more nervous. It was an eerie feeling standing in the dim light trying to adjust our eyes into an interior that was cast in evening shades.

Just as we started to peer in, a chicken flew out the door, squawking and flapping. My heart stopped beating and I could tell I wasn't breathing. Then from somewhere in the room came a voice called out, "Is that you, Sr. Carol?"

"Good Lord, Leonard, you 'bout scared us to death! Why in the world are you sitting here in the dark? Where is your lamp, and I'll light it for you."

"No, I will," he said, striking a wooden match against a brick lying on the floor beside him without getting up. "I was sitting here watching the sun go down." And leaning over the lantern, applied the match to the wick and the room slowly brightened, as the air dampened with the scent of kerosene.

When he adjusted the wick, I was able to have my first glimpse of Leonard. He had the rugged face typical of a Native American with a strong jaw with no mustache or beard (*unable to grow this false machismo, Indians sport bare chins*) with a dark tan with deep laugh lines around his eyes revealing his face had taken some long hours in the intensely dry New Mexico sun.

I was introduced out of courtesy but I held about as much interest for Leonard as if I were selling vacuums, but if chickens pecked insects from his dirt floor, he already had his vacuuming covered. Small talk was not Leonard's strong suit as I watched Sr. Carol and Leonard exchange community news, Carol doing most of the talking. With his feet crossed in front of him, Leonard was content just to sit and listen. I admired his lack of jabber and was taken by his contemplative nature as he leaned back in his worn comfortable arm chair.

I asked myself the question, wasn't this what I had been striving for in the monastery? Renunciation of the world and renunciation of self? In very undramatic ways I realized Leonard had achieved detachment and real peace. Did this simple one room hogan with an old rusty pipe sticking up through a hole in the roof act like a hermitage just as it did for Thomas Merton? Was Leonard actually sitting in the light of his own consciousness? What was wrong watching the world go by listening to the constant drone of crickets, a hesychast would ask? It takes real contentment such as Leonard's to prove Browning's point, "God's in His heaven and all is right with the world." As I looked at the mixture of dented pots and pans along a shelf on the wall and the water barrel he used as a wood stove, I felt the force of his circumstances like scavenging wolves sliding through a forest of pine.

It was the eleventh hour when we finally said goodnight, leaving Leonard as we had found him, sitting motionless in his big chair in total presence, staring straight ahead, yet seemingly less moribund after getting to know him. Waving Yah-te-hey from our car windows, I swayed to the left as our car bolted into motion. It made me think about the severity and duration of the rough ride we had ahead. Squaring my shoulders, I hung on for dear life.

On the ride out, I thought Sr. Carol must have been maintaining her speed while we talked, after all I had only just met her. The ride back was a different story. I was a little concerned when we gained air hurtling a hole. My concern wasn't entirely unfounded as I remembered how vision problems acted up in people who had MS. What could come from all this bouncing and jarring? It had to have an effect. I calmed myself as I remembered the line that patients having early attacks involving vision problems usually recover fully."[6] I put my faith in that sentence and steadied myself by holding on to the dashboard, hoping they were right. Could it knock my eyes back into nystagmus, when my eyes were jumping around? Or bring back another bout of nausea, anything but that, I thought, while we turned onto a road deep in the reservation.

Realizing she had a captive audience in the seat beside her and not wanting to blow a golden opportunity of saving my immortal soul, Sr. Carol began sharing a series of warnings and impending chastisements doomed for the earth if we, as sinners, didn't straighten up and become remorseful.

"The justice of God will fall like a thunderbolt," she began quoting the stigmatist Sr. Aiello. (A genuine stigmatist is one who bears the bleeding wounds of Christ on their body.) Needless to say, this is not the best topic for conversation explaining how the earth will experience episodes of darkness and firestorms during the *Three Days of Darkness*.[7] Why would she bring this up now when it was so dark I could hardly make out the road we were driving on.

"Steady as she goes," Sr. Carol calmed, feeling my head lightly hit the roof.

"I'm all right," I reassured, hoping my vision would be too. She had no idea between her impending "1800 thunderstorms," to the power struggle with my eyes, and the car sickness I was ignoring in my stomach, I was doing everything to hold myself together and keep working properly, while wondering how much more I could take. Since my walking hadn't given me away with poor coordination or a loss of balance, there was no reason to mention I had MS, so I never had.

Seeing me as another soul to save, Sr. Carol didn't want to waste valuable road time, so kept up the pace of frightening judgments and prophecies: "Fight ye children of light; combat, ye small band that can see!" (Our lady of LaSalette), so by the time we finally shot up the hill to the retreat between the harrowing ride and worrying about whether I had already been corrupted, and worrying about my health, this was not the best topic for conversation on the way back to the retreat. When I was dropped off in front of the Brother Sun hogan, I wanted to get out and kiss the ground. I opened the car door and when the exit light came on, I turned my face so she couldn't see if my face had turned green from the ride; not from car sickness, but from worry.

In a commanding tone, I heard one last "Praise Jesus!" as she turned the Bronco around and sped off into the darkness, still trying to convince me to turn my life around as well.

After I locked the door of my hogan behind me, I checked my vision first thing. I flicked on the lights and looked directly at St. Francis's poem hanging on the wall and used it like an eye chart; "Praise be to thee..." my optic nerve was fine and holding steady "...with all Thy creatures." I concluded my eyes were no worse for wear, and I could start trusting my body would hold up under adverse conditions, besides, for peace of mind, I carried the nausea pills with me always. My balance seemed to be all right too, as I walked down the hall to my bedroom. I realized that between the yard work and trips to the reservation, I told myself it was good to be guarded, but not overly cautious.

After changing into my pajamas, I crawled into bed. As per my usual routine, I pulled the curtains to the side at the corner and watched the agitated lights move restlessly over the city. I thought back to Leonard. I remembered watching from the car window until the darkness swallowed him up and wondered why he didn't just lower the wick instead of snuffing it out completely. Preferring to sit in the darkness, maybe he was watching the lights in the night like I was.

I thought of Sr. Carol, glory be to God! and wondered if she had ever given Leonard the same overview of the Day of Wrath she had given me, not with the intention of frightening him, but to enlighten him. If this were the case, it would explain his reticence for he too may have been determining, that with Sr. Carol, "It is good to be guarded, but not overly cautious."

I lay in total darkness fighting to keep my eyes open as I listened to the sound of the crickets chirping outside, but still awake enough to hear the incidental end of a lyric run effortlessly through my mind:

> Cold-hearted orb that rules the night
> Removes the colors from our sight,
> Red is gray and yellow white
> But we decide which is right,
> And which is an illusion.[8]

There was no illusion about this though, Leonard and I had a lot in common.

Chapter 10—Typecast

The impact of last night's ride faded from my memory like a dream of a white buffalo lost in a dust cloud.

Yawning, I reached for the cord to pull open the drapes next to my bed and looked away as bright light flooded the hogan. After a time my eyes landed on a long-legged mosquito clinging to a trunk of a pine tree, the insect's narrow disjointed legs tightly hugging the tree. I studied its delicate net-veined wings and long slender body as it rested quietly on the outer covering of bark, indulging its long proboscis in a welcome lull as though it had landed on a puddle of sugar water.

In contrast, my eyes moved to a slow moving beetle similar to a carpet beetle. It was carrying a hard brown shell on its back stoically climbing over pine needles and small rocks, up and down, never slowing, confident in its steady progress. Scavenging roots, wood, leaves and flowers hunting down prey as masterly as a tiger.

Dressing, I thought there must be a better way to wake up than focusing on insects first thing in the morning. I didn't see the car on my walk over, Hyacinth must have gotten up and out early. And as I scooped the last bit of cereal into my spoon I looked out the Retreat Center's small dining room off the kitchen at the patches of brown weeds covering the hills below. There was nothing stirring, not even a bird, as I stopped crunching a moment to appreciate the quiet.

The roar of a truck making a fast track up the hill outside made me jump. Probably an Indian coming up to fill a water barrel, I guessed. But when I didn't hear the familiar clanging of the empty container against sides of the truck, I knew I had visitors.

I picked up my bowl and spoon and carried it to the kitchen to clean and when I looked out the window, I saw it was only Sr. Hyacinth. As I dried the bowl I noticed she wasn't alone, she had two passengers: one barely able to see over the dashboard, and the other barely had enough clearance for her head. All three were wearing black veils!

With Sr. Hyacinth leading the way they walked to the door and into the kitchen. "Hi Anne. Bet you think these are sisters from a bordering parish? They're not our neighbors, they're novices! *Our* novices," she said, happy her community had obliged her with the extra help.

Hyacinth hadn't said anything about their arrival in preparation, a trait I was learning to accept, and I was at a loss for words. That's when the tall one introduced herself. "I'm Sr. Godwina, Godwin for short," glad she hadn't gone with the shorter version still. Looking down at me from her tall frame, I could see she was even wearing flat sandals.

"I'm Sr. Evangelista," the shorter one piped in and shook my hand in greeting, and as she looked up at me, I thought her name was taller than she was. She had a smattering of dark freckles across the bridge of her nose and was wearing very sturdy light colored shoes which matched her sturdy legs. I've never known a good cook who wasn't carrying their tasting in a few extra pounds, and little Sr. Evangelista was no exception.

Sr. Hyacinth raised an index finger and said, "These two energetic Sisters from one of our other retreat centers volunteered to help us here at St. Francis and Celeste at the girl's home. Sr. Godwina has a few psychology classes under her belt, and Sr. Evangelista is a cook and has a few meals under her belt as well," Sr. Hyacinth said, smiling. "I know we'll be able to use both."

"Wait till you try my cornbread," Evangelista prodded. "The trick is to make several shallow, diagonal slices across the top with a single edge razor blade to keep the crusts from cracking," nodding her head with conviction.

She really knows her breads, I thought, picturing the kitchen littered with baking sheets and paper muffin cups from this experienced retreat cook.

"But I'm more known for my pastries," she continued, smiling wide as she fancied herself a pastry chef. "Cakes turnovers, scones, and fritters."

"We can use all the help we can get," I said enthusiastically as I saw my work load cut drastically with the arrival of these two co-workers in their twenties. It made a big difference that they were experienced and knew retreat work could be fast and furious and not so much lotus eating.

"They'll be staying in two of the extra bedrooms in the retreat which we shall now officially call a convent. It will be nice having Sisters to say the Office with in the chapel (daily recitation of psalms and prayers)."

"Come on, everyone grab a suitcase and I'll show them to their rooms so they can get settled in. We'll meet back here for coffee and a snack afterwards."

Hallways in convents were always the same, dim and colorless, maybe a picture of a sacred painting hanging at eye level, plastic night lights running the length of the hall elucidating the darkness instead of expensive light fixtures giving the impression comfortless bedrooms were behind the closed doors.

Walking along the airless corridor, I suddenly found myself in my thoughts walking down the passageway in the monastery and it wouldn't have surprised me in the least to have bumped into the Sister who had been in charge of the art department there. It wasn't until I returned to Sr. Evangelista's room to drop off an extension cord and found her happily straightening the twin bedspread around her half-emptied suitcase, and saw a clock already displaying the correct time placed on the pine desk, and her shoes neatly placed in pairs in rows arranged in the closet under a few hanging white short-sleeved blouses that it hit me, "My God, she is like the worker beetle!"

Passing by Sr. Godwina's room I had to refrain from checking her arms for spider-like veins. At a glance in her room I saw she either was a practicing minimalist, which, when I thought about it, is what religious were anyway, or she had been raised to be happy and content with few possessions and going without and making do was perfectly acceptable for her.

Like the insects, both Sisters exhibited her own unique personality. Rubbing my chin as I walked by the two rooms to the kitchen, that's when one of the most unique weeks I spent in the monastery came back to me in a rush. 'Examining an hypothesis' I think that's how the student explained it. Even if her question is not verbalized, most people think they know the answer already (including me); aren't all cloistered Sisters the same type?

And in my mind, I was back in the community room at the monastery listening to a psychology student from the University of Tucson.

The student, working towards her doctorate, obtained special permission to conduct a test using contemplative Sisters. I had never heard of the *Myers-Briggs Type Indicator* test of personalities before but her supposition was that every one in our monastery would be basically the same type. What she learned added another year of work to her thesis![9]

Approximately thirty years old, the grad student began by giving us an explication of her experiment, to see what type of personalities we had. Our desks had been arranged in a large circle and at each place was a small packet of papers face down. I guessed that the preconceived notion she had about us most was that of introverted, bookworm types.

"Classifying and defining differences will help you get along better and be more patient with each other. Understanding how others communicate and knowing where they're coming from, you can utilize it in your dealings with each other," was how the student persuaded us the test was worth taking. She explained how the Myers-Briggs Type Indicator test used initials from the words Introvert, Intuitive, Feeler, Perceiver and a combination of these initials will help to classify our true image. "And don't worry, if you're not pleased with the traits you exhibit now, in time they generally change and evolve, for example an introvert will become more extroverted, and so forth."

"That's a bit of good news anyway," the superior said. "For a moment there, I thought our traits would grow, especially the bad ones." We all breathed a communal sigh of relief.

On that note, the student asked us to turn over the papers in front of us and begin.

I have always been a good test-taker, not letting my nerves get the better of me, not blanking out or becoming sick with worry, and the fact that we weren't being graded, and there was no pressure made this test easy to take.

Two weeks later after she had gone over our tests, I can still picture the growing redness on the grad student's face. I can still hear her incredulous cry: "I can't believe it! If I hadn't checked it with my own eyes, I never would have believed it!" I can still hear her cry, "Not one out of the thirteen is the same. You're all different!"

I understood why she was so emotional. What she discovered was something completely different than what she based years of hard work on. The image of her throwing her dissertation out the window with her shredded hypothesis behind it came to mind.

Her findings were amazing really, and something she could spend another year discussing in her new treatise. To think we had extroverts mixed in our community with introverts, loud mouths with the closed lipped, non-conforming Sisters with the conventional, realists in with the dreamers, logical personalities together with the irrational. But what stood out most in my mind, and I hoped the graduate student realized this too, was the amazing fact with all our differences, *we were all able to get along!*[10]

All this rushed through my mind as I walked along the dim hallway in the Retreat house leading to the small dining room where I found Sr. Hyacinth precisely cutting up a loaf of date-nut bread. Unselfish in her giving and liberal with her portions, she asked me to join her.

"Care for some cream cheese with your bread?" she urged, pushing a dish of soft white cheese toward me.

As generous with her time as she was the sizes, I eagerly accepted. I *knew* she would ask me to join her while we waited for our new colleagues. "Don't mind if I do," I said with a smile, because she was just that type.

Chapter 11—Lucked Out

New Mexico nights are chilly, especially at elevated heights over 5,000 feet. I lay in my bed in my hogan with the blankets and counterpane pulled up close around my neck thinking back on Leonard and wondering how he was managing with his door off. I was enveloped in a feeling of disbelief at how incredibly lucky I was to have actually been inside an authentic hogan and meeting an authentic Indian. It made me think back to another time when at the monastery I had this same overwhelming feeling of being lucky.

It was during a celebration of a Silver Jubilarian, but it wasn't the run of the mill celebration with tablecloths, cheese and wine, rites, readings and rejoicing. I had volunteered to help with the seating arrangements but I wanted to do it with a fun twist. I would let each Sister pull out the first half of a Scripture quote from a vase, and wherever she found the finish of the quote, that's where she'd sit. To liven it up, I tried to pick 12 quotes that were fresh and not too commonplace. The problem was I chose quotes that were way too obscure like: "When I kept silent, my bones grew old through my groaning all the day long. For night and day your hand was heavy upon me;…my vitality was turned into the drought of summer." And, "Before your thorns harden and grow, changing from tender thorns into a thick hedge and shutting out the sight of God as even oft-times the living find their thread of life broken in the midst of its course…even so will God swallow them up in the midst of His wrath."

What started out to be a parlor game ended up with everyone walking around and around the long refectory table bumping into one another, scratching their heads, racking their brains trying to find their matching quote so they could sit down in this game of spiritual musical chairs. Because I'd made the quotes way too difficult, it was amusing. What's worse, because I knew the end of my quote I was the only one able to be seated so I ended up watching this parade of spirituality diligently searching and circling as they made their way round and round the table.

I relished my incredible luck. I knew even then I was privileged to be able to see into a way of life closed to most people during this once-in-a-lifetime celebration, and I also knew the importance wasn't in the good food and wine, but in the camaraderie I felt with the community. I didn't hear one vulgar expression made out of frustration, in fact, because this was a contemplative community and they had taken a vow of silence, no one said anything. All I heard were the swishing of their habits as they passed again and again, soft chimes from the clock in the hall as it struck the hour, and the intermittent cawing of a disturbed crow outside.

After what seemed an interminable amount of time, everyone was finally seated. Glancing down the long distance to the very end of the wooden table, I saw the disgruntled face of the Novice Mistress sitting among the lowly unprofessed novices, and realized sometimes in life it *is* just the luck of the draw.

Tucked away in my hogan, I must have been hiding my imperfections still because I involuntarily pulled the covers up over my head as I remembered, and giggled myself to sleep.

Chapter 12—The Dichotomy of a Pow Wow

"They called it a Pow Wow," Sr. Evangelista exclaimed loudly. "A spiritual ceremony celebrating the spirit world of their ancestors. At least that's what the girls told me. 'It's held in the spring, to celebrate new life,' is what they said."

Poor Sr. Evangelista looked and sounded depleted in the aftermath.

"Sister, kids would have told you the pope was making an appearance to get you to go along," I empathized in return, referring to the teens at the home.

To Native Americans who are used to Pow Wows and grew up attending these events, I bet they are blasé, but to someone like Sr. Evangelista new to the Southwest, the gathering must have shocked her sensibilities; a true culture shock.

"But what was it like?" I asked, genuinely interested. I had heard these festivals were times to help keep traditional ways of Indians alive by helping people, participants and spectators, understand the importance of the role tradition plays in their lives.

"Well, everyone seemed to know everyone else. It was like one big tribal party," Sister blurted out. "There were booths selling souvenirs, crafts, supplies and food. Ruby kept pestering me for change for cherry drinks the whole time."

"Was there dancing?"

"Yes, continual dancing. Everybody danced."

"Did you dance?"

She looked at me with raised eyes and moved her dark framed glasses back up on her nose and decisively said, "No, no, I didn't but the girls did. The girls were hard to keep track of, I kept losing sight of them. Some of the dances were sacred I was told, and were danced in a special area."

"What were they wearing?"

"Oh that's another thing. Everyone was in traditional Navajo dress, long colorful fringes, feathers, really striking outfits, and here I was in my black habit and veil not blending in very well at all."

"That must mean there was music?"

"Music? Was there music?" she repeated herself, her eyes growing big, almost crossing in alarm. "It never stopped. Anne, the entire Pow Wow lasted five hours and I don't think there was a second that didn't have drums beating! Boom boom boom! I tell you I think I may have suffered permanent hearing loss!"

"I see," I commiserated while watching her place a palm of her hand against her right ear tapping it gently to test it.

"Boom boom boom," she imitated again. "If they were trying to wake ancestral spirits, I think they succeeded. Boom boom boom," she said as she wiped her wet brow.

"I see," I said, letting her get it out of her system. It must have been a blessed relief to be away from the drumming, the quiet at the retreat acting like balm on her frazzled nerves.

She stopped for a moment and regrouped her thoughts.

"You know the whole Pow Wow really is an impressive Navajo experience you shouldn't miss," suddenly building it up.

"I know, but you said…"

"There's another one in three days. Sr. Celeste and I will be taking the girls again. Do you want to go with us?

She must have noticed the dumbfounded expression on my face and knew I needed more convincing. So reaching into one of the deep pockets of her habit, she pulled out a small object.

Dangling the woven container under my nose like a bribe, she said with a twisted smile, "Look, you can buy a basket!"

Chapter 13—Old World Birds

The scent of a skunk's organic release wafting silently through the creases between the timbers of my walls in my hogan brought me to full wakefulness. It wasn't a sudden awakening but a slow questioning insistence starting with '*what* is that *smell?*" And mashing my nose against a pillow, a fearful 'is it *in* the house?' It wasn't a nauseating odor, just a very strong one, like walking into an enclosed hen house on a hot day. It begged the question: *how can a smell wake me up?*

It made me reflect on whether the scent was actually *in* my mouth. I reminded myself again that a strong scent left by an animal was much better than one left by an unnatural chemical odor or smelling toxic emissions left by the audibility of traffic giving off noise as well as emissions. Considering this was the day I had set aside to go on a hike to study the world in the serenity of nature and all its phenomena, stinky or otherwise, I couldn't have asked for a better start to my day than being awakened by nature's alarm clock.

One thing I knew for sure; they weren't vultures. I had watched these large birds in circular cavalcades soaring on the winds, their broad strong wings wide open in soaring flights. They were gravitating toward a certain hill, and I wanted to see why. Following their flight on the ground by running along underneath was nearly impossible as they covered so much distance, and I had to deal with stumbling over rocks and crevasses while they had unlimited flying space that covered from here to China. This was the challenge, to track them through indefinite space.

New Mexico terrain is similar to Arizona terrain with its buttes and crags and hot, dry weather. But as I walked I began to see differences between the two; the soil in New Mexico had an overwhelmingly reddish hue very noticeable in the sides of cliffs, and although Arizona has spectacular rock formations, nothing could compare to the balancing acts of rock based on pillar-like columns of stones atop huge boulders, which in turn, balanced ill-proportioned shapes twice their size. It took centuries of eroding winds to fashion these fantastic monolithic shapes that appeared to be indissoluble while managing to avoid the very winds that could topple them.

The hill I was walking on led down into a cleared basin and up another hill, and in this up and down trajectory I kept looking up at the sky to see if I still had the birds in sight. More often then not, I would lose them only to have them reappear out of nowhere, almost as if they knew I was following them, and wanted me to.

I stopped to admire a species of cactus I had never seen before. It was bespangled with large open red flowers like someone had encircled a ruby necklace around the entire barrel of the globular cactus. It had unbranched ribbed spiny stems as sharp as needles so I couldn't get close enough to the flowers to detect a scent, but admiring it from afar, it was breathtaking. I wouldn't want to accidentally fall into its clutches, but I had to admire its survival ploy that used a sequin of red flowers to attract birds that had kept the species growing for eons. I walked around and around the leafless plant admiring its numerous cactus flowers.

I couldn't imagine robins coming anywhere near this spiny cactus (nimble-footed hummingbirds, maybe). I made a point to remember the place and would definitely come back to it when I took these fauna and flora nature hikes. After this short flower interlude, I went back looking for the birds.

Not a bird watcher by nature, I tried to figure out what kind of birds I was following by a process of elimination. I knew what owls looked like, and these were not owls. Besides, owls seldom flew in the daytime. They certainly weren't pigeons. Maybe they were magpies, but I didn't know what a magpie looked like. Too small for eagles and they didn't have the white heads associated with eagles. Maybe they were falcons, or hawks? No, a soaring hawk was easy to distinguish. Or could they be ravens? I'd never heard the croaking call of a raven before so I had nothing to go on. I knew what crows looked like, were familiar with their calls. I knew the phrase, "jackdaw in peacock's feathers" meant a deceiver, jackdaw describing a species of crow. The birds I was chasing from afar did seem to have the glossy blackness associated with crows.

As I was looking up at them from a distance, I almost walked into a three wire fence running east to west that must have been separating ranch land from other property. I gave a tentative and somewhat guilty look around and crawled through. I continued walking and came upon several large red rocks sticking out of the ground. Not resisting this chance for some unchallenging rock climbing, I clambered over them only because they were so beautifully shaped; odd, but beautiful in their coarse contours, running my hands over their forms in appreciation. Drawing myself up to full height, I jumped off the middle one and went back to tracking the birds.

Cutting my way across the hill around little scrub bushes and cactus, I noticed my walking had become easier on this gradual, but steady, uphill climb. The ground was more solidly packed and there were less botanicals dressing the ground to walk around so I didn't have to be as careful.

After making good headway, I suddenly pulled up and stopped. There before me was a view so magnificent it took my breath away. Many hundreds of miles away I could see an incredibly long and narrow mountain range stretching north and south that had clouds nestled on both ends giving it a ground-less look of a dream. It didn't have the usual high mountain peaks but looked as if it was edged with imposing block-like ledges. Almost eye level at this distance, sporadic coverings of slow moving clouds gave the impression it was moving in and out of the atmosphere with an 'out of this world' quality. It truly was breathtaking; all I wanted to do was sit where I was in the dirt and admire this long horizontal stratum on a parallel mountain far away as a feeling of insignificance flooded my being.

Unable to pull my eyes away, I stayed and gazed at this commanding panoramic view for about an hour, slowly following the ever changing patchwork of colors cast by the clouds. Hearing psalm 27 in my head, up here it was easy to heed its command to wait. I was aware the continental divide separated river systems making them flow in opposite directions east or west but I didn't think I would ever be lucky enough to observe it with my own eyes. Was I this close? What else could it be? I then remembered reading a brochure in the conference room at the retreat about an ice cave. It talked about an expanse of land considered to be *the* most moon-like terrain on all the earth with a trail leading into a collapsed lava tube. Its temperature never rose above 31 degrees. Reading on, I remembered it was only 72 miles from Gallup at an elevation of 8,000 feet, but was I up that high?

Out of nowhere one of the birds I was following, now down to one, flew directly across my line of vision and interrupted my wordless watching with unhurried flapping. It let out a loud *caw* in greeting, breaking the silence like an angry cry of a cat, hoping to hear a vocal mimicry response. Unmoved, it loosely flapped its wings in scoff, allowing me to see glints of deep blue and purple on its feathers, and continued flying. Seeing it up close I knew now for sure it was of the crow species. After ditching the others, I felt this wasn't an ordinary crow being able to endure intense quiet and aloneness. With noble qualities such as these, I guessed it to be an old world crow. And remembering what Thomas Merton had written reminded me I was in good stead: "The chief function of monastic silence is then to preserve that *memoria Dei* which is much more than "memory." It is a total consciousness and awareness of God which is impossible without silence, recollection and a certain withdrawal" (*Cistercian Life*, 1974). It was all the proof I needed.

From then on the continental divide represented a division between speech and silence for me, and I made sure when I visited this awe-inspiring place, I would leave my words at the base of the hill and adapt the language of listening needed for waiting, inside and out. The clouds made it easy to do, for I was already out of myself just by looking at the view. Each break in the faraway clouds was like a real presence of clarity and I felt transfigured even without the presence of bell, book or candle.

Where was it off to now? Assuring myself the Great Divide would still be here if I left, I looked around at the few rocks and scanty bunches of grass, and ran my hand across the dirt in homage like a meaningful end to a rite. Climbing to my feet I trekked down the backside of the hill in a walk-trot, stopping every so often to catch my breath with deep gulps of air and to admire the mountain range that seemed to go on forever.

Coming down a different side I reached the bottom of the hill on level footing and saw a very different topography of innumerable hill tops dissolving in the distance surrounded by vistas of sun covered fields. Split river beds, dry and knocked flat, splintered the region's floor like a bedspread, and noticed land formations that were more severely sculpted bluffs with broad fronts.

I located the bird skimming its way carelessly through the sky and watched as it flew back and forth for some time, almost like it was pacing. And as I twisted around and looked up, I saw why. Situated on top the next hill, like a castle, was a rock formation of considerable magnitude held up by a sheer vertical cliff that was streaked with long vertical stains from years of sliding wind and rain and dirt. About three-quarters of the way up, I could see between twenty and thirty holes, like miniature caves, curving around the hill that looked to have been there for centuries. They were so high I couldn't reach them if I wanted to, and besides, the cliff face was convexly angled in such a way, it looked top heavy slanting the steep precipice outward the higher it went. The bird had a great place for waiting!

Convinced its nest was safe from unwelcome intruders, the crow flew up to a hole, slowing its speed with aeronautical precision almost to a float, and entered one of the selected nests in the colony. It disappeared briefly only to stick its head out with a message of *caw, caw, caw*. Soon a small flock assembled in a gathered flying.

It didn't take long for the air above me above me to be filled with milling crows and scolding calls. I decided to vacate the nest area because from my vantage point looking up from bottom to top, it didn't take long for my neck and shoulders to begin to feel tight and strained. I was surprised to find crows perched in rocks, but I suppose concealing themselves in this special hiding place made sense; high enough to watch for predators and for food, clever enough to take advantage of these ready-made roosts, but most importantly it was a great place to wait undisturbed.

I felt my familiar tinge of excitement when I at last took off exploring again not hampered by following the birds, feeling the spirits of Indians more clearly the deeper in I walked. I know it was my imagination but it felt like Indian spirits were escorting me through the five periods of Native American culture I'd read about—Archaic, Basketmaker, Anastazi, Hopi and Navajo epochs.

With the landscape leveling out into low-lying hillocks, I found myself walking on someone else's trail which could have easily been here 2500 BC I convinced myself, half-expecting an Indian to jump from behind a bush. But nothing eventful happened until…as I continued on the path through hilly mounds of rust colored earth flanked by low ridges of darker soil, I was totally surprised when the trail led to an exciting find—a small pond! This pristine and quiet pool surrounded by olive-green stalks and reeds gleaming brightly in the late afternoon sun, was teeming with insects and an occasional small fish or frog feeding off its transparent false bottom scattering the water.

Not believing what I was seeing, I stooped to touch it for myself letting the cold water drip from my fingers back into the water. On an impulse, I looked up into the sky and saw that I had been trailed, by the crow! Now it was following me, and I watched as its reflection flashed across the glassy surface of the pond.

The scent from a pond is different from a running stream or a babbling brook, a standing fresh body of water has a scent-less odor, but for the chlorophyll from the green pigments in the surrounding weeds. Undefiled by motors and noise and people, this land-locked sheet of water had a timeless scent of purity and cleanliness, and I felt cleansed just inhaling.

Thinking of how I started the day brought back a bad taste to my mouth, skunk. I sucked in as much of the pure pond air as I could and knew the end of this day was substantially better than its beginning.

Skimming the banks with my eyes, I caught the eyes of the crow that had landed and waded in, splashing as it preened, ducking its head under a couple of times, dipping its bill, then raising it, taking several drinks before finally resting, both of us sunning ourselves in a 'hurry-up and wait attitude' doing nothing, deferring action to allow the passage of time to work in our favor.

It was a nice way to end my nature walk, I thought, waving good-bye. I couldn't think of better company to have as a fellow *waiter*; the jackdaw and me, two old world birds.

Chapter 14—The People

"Did you walk here with The Great Spirit?" Sr. Hyacinth asked, trying to find some common ground with the stranger.

"Yeah," he answered flatly…"but I got my truck parked just up the hill," throwing a thumb out towards the top of the hill.

This was Franklin. At this example of Navajo logic, I looked at Hyacinth and saw the corners of her eyes tightening as she tried to disguise a smile at this unique blend of traditional and modern beliefs. "If you're here looking for work, we can use a man with a truthful spirit.

"I am, and I haven't had a drink in over a month," he volunteered with pride.

"Good. If you want to work here, keep it that way," Hyacinth said straightforwardly, her tone changing from happenstance encounter to businesswoman. "I'll have none of that at the retreat."

Franklin was a funny little man. I first saw him standing in the retreat yard leaning against the statue of Jesus, bent over, cleaning the heals of his boots with a stick. Usually Navajos don't want anything to do with the dead, so I guessed he didn't know who he was propped up against or he knew spirits could never be contained in hard plaster.

Franklin's bent posture bolted upright on hearing Sr. Hyacinth's heavy footsteps plodding across the yard toward him with introductions imminent.

"Yah te hey Sister," I heard him say meekly, noticing as he straightened up how much he was dwarfed by Hyacinth's height and girth.

"Yah te hey," she greeted, both of us sizing up the little man about fifty, age being determined by charm and vitality rather than looks, for guessing a Navajo's age was tricky; crippled and toothless could be signs of a rough life and not necessarily of the elderly. My guesses were usually off about twenty years, either way. This time was no exception; Franklin was thirty.

Like others who have wandered into the retreat looking for work or a square meal, she knew from experience that alcohol was a serious problem on the community and in the city of Gallup and wasn't to be taken lightly.

"I am a good worker and I work hard," sidestepping her message of reform.

"Be here tomorrow and I'll have work for you. Bring gloves if you have them. Anne here will show you what to do," bidding him good bye.

I felt I was standing on the wrong side of a wall because I had no idea what Hyacinth was talking about, and this work she had for Franklin, no doubt, was going to include me. All I knew was it involved gloves.

Franklin's arrival was fortunate timing, and if I hadn't known better, I would have thought a friendly informant in town had slipped him the contents of a delivery invoice, because when Tuesday arrived, so did Franklin and then the dump trucks. Three trucks worth, hauling durable, waterproof, plum-pink colored rocks, cubic yards of the stuff, each truck dumping their loads in the retreat yard.

I didn't have to wait long before Sr. Hyacinth appeared giving commands, her shouting drowned in the motorized lifting of the truck beds jerking and shifting, trying to slide the rocks off the beds of the trucks. Then fastening the stiff open flaps back in place on the heavy-duty trucks, they were gone leaving three large piles of loose labor in the yard.

When the dust settled, I walked to the closest pile and picked up a rock. Odd color, I thought turning it over in my fingers. It looked very similar to a piece of volcanic lava, except the color, very porous and abrasive (I wouldn't want to fall on it) and heavy. The piece I was holding in my palm felt as heavy as a large fishing weight.

"Won't this be better instead of mud and snow for the retreatants to walk on? We'll have stone paths all around the retreat center!" smiling appreciatively.

"They are a lot of nice rocks," I said to Hyacinth as an understatement, who, by the gratified look on her face, was already picturing the elegance of beautiful stone walks connecting the retreat hall and chapel with all the hogans.

At the moment I wasn't concerned with how they would enhance the center. I was thinking of the work involved to complete her design scheme.

"Franklin, I want these rocks to go on these paths," the director instructed, pointing to the paths that were leading directly to hogans. "Anne will show you."

True to his word, early the next day Franklin showed up holding an old pair of gloves. And I was only too happy to show him what to do, I wouldn't have missed it for the world because I hoped I would be able to pick up insightful bits of information about things Navajo, past and present. Whereas Leonard, sitting alone on the reservation wasn't much of a talker, I couldn't get Franklin to stop talking. In between his trips dumping wheelbarrows of the pink quarry stones, I was lucky enough to hear first-hand about the Indian culture.

I didn't know that Navajos were taught never eat food that has the point of a knife in it. And because they are warned against killing snakes I made a special mental note never to tell about the snakes I had to kill in Arizona.

Listening to Franklin I learned Navajos were taught to stay away from trees damaged by lightening, noting to myself again never to bring up I was in a monastery that was struck by a large bolt of lightening damaging the electrical system, but we continued living in the cloisters even while the hallways were still smoky. I wouldn't bring it up in conversation with him.

Or how the Navajo religion didn't believe souls of the dead belonged to an afterlife, but thought the evil part of a dead person stayed on earth in the form of *chindi*, spirits that returned to the place where the person died to haunt the living. Adjusting his grip on the handles of the wheelbarrow, Franklin warned in all seriousness possibly to ward off any lingering *chindi*, "One should avoid *chindi* at all costs!"

I didn't bring it up how this belief reminded me of what St. John of the Cross wrote about how evils torment and afflict souls when they are bound to their desires, (*Ascent of Mount Carmel*, Chapter XII), but I was thinking it.

I learned the Navajo people referred to themselves as the *Dineh,* meaning *the people,* and because of this they "…had no choice but to follow a narrow path through a world swarming with supernatural beings. Powerless creatures such as humans could survive only by learning to live in harmony with these forces."[9] This belief sounded vaguely familiar as I saw similarities to 'walking the narrow path,' following ancient monastic traditions teeming with saints, and how the powerless novice will survive only by learning to live in harmony with forces that had gone before.

Franklin continued hauling wheelbarrows of the small pink rock over the yard, emptying them a little at a time on the paths as I pushed and settled them evenly on the walkways with a rake. By listening to his accounts and explanations to his stories, I uncovered meanings behind the apparent ones. Not knowing what to believe, I weighed the practical against the possible, and decided this was how it was always going to be with Franklin.

"You know, the Inter-Tribal Ceremonial parade has passed, but another one is coming up," Franklin coaxed. "If you really are want to know about the Navajo, you should come see our parade."

"I'll ask Sr. Hyacinth," I said, but wondering what attending a parade could teach me.

"You will learn many things," he replied, reading my mind.

The next day I couldn't wait for Franklin to arrive so I could tell him the good news. We would attend the Christmas parade with Srs. Hyacinth and Celeste and the girls in Gallup. The Sisters thought it was important for the group home girls to connect with their heritage, it was an annual outing for them.

The week went by with Franklin shoveling and me raking, but I could tell there was something on his mind. He didn't divulge any more information about what was so special about seeing the parade, other than there would be the usual floats and school marching bands playing Christmas carols. I was sure it was going to be another typical public procession with participants showing off their marching skills.

We had leveled one rock pile so far. With two more to go, I looked at the dim sky with anxiety. Not because of what rain could do to our work turning the unused piles sodden mounds weighing as much as concrete, and not because rain could bring the parade to a standstill. I was anxious about how a change in the weather might affect my MS. Did cold weather affect people with MS as much as heat? If heat worsened symptoms in some people with MS even by taking hot baths, would cold weather do the same? It was one thing to exert energy and body warmth doing physical labor but quite another lollygagging on a street corner for hours in cold weather watching a slow-moving parade go by, and tomorrow was parade day.

I didn't say anything about my misgivings to Franklin or Sr. Hyacinth of course. I was worried because I remembered reading that the highest incidence of MS in the world was in Scotland, and Scotland has bitterly cold winters. Does this mean cold weather exacerbates MS symptoms, or was it the lack of sunshine at the increased latitude that causes MS symptoms to flair up? Keeping these concerns to myself, I prepared to meet the cold head on. How else was I going to know how far I could push myself except by using my body like a barometer; if I collapsed in the street due to paralysis, I would definitely know to stay out of the cold.

Franklin must have noticed my distracted sky watching because he said, "No snow," making me wonder how he could say that with such confidence.

The next day, wearing thermals under my jeans, a green coat with sheepskin lining, black mittens and my old red knitted ski hat pulled over my ears, I checked to make sure a half pill for nausea was in my pocket. I was ready to brave the elements, and oh yes, to see the parade.

Drifting in from every direction was a good cross section of Gallup's population lining the parade route and I wondered if every Navajo there had prepared a small bag of medicine, like Franklin talked about, to protect him when he was among strangers. Who is say if part of a liver from an animal or corn pollen carried in a pouch wouldn't help? Maybe embracing a belief will actually make it happen, wasn't I doing the same thing in taking control of my emotional well-being by believing nothing more was going to happen to me physically as long as I carried the small pouch of pills?

Waving to Ruby on the other side of street, I saw Sr. Celeste with the group home girls in a front row position. Small Sr. Evangelista was there claiming a front spot as well, helping Celeste keep a watchful eye on the girls, mindful no one would be accidentally pushed into the street during the parade. Sr. Hyacinth and myself with the tall Sr. Godwina standing behind us, both wearing their long black Franciscan habits, kept our heads turned down the street hoping to see movement from the oncoming step-by-step procession.

"Here they come!" I heard Ruby yell excitedly as she leaned into the street.

School bands led the way with cheerleaders twirling batons with only a few minor contretemps slowing the parade in its tracks as a baton was picked up, checked for damage, and returned to its original twirling gyrations. In a small town like Gallup, there weren't many high schools and this section went by quickly.

Philanthropic groups carried banners announcing the name of their group, and educational foundations passed by with medium sized followings. There were several Indian sponsored programs and banners displaying names of mission schools; next in line were two battered women's programs behind a 'needy family' organization. There was one alcohol counseling center with only two parade participants each carrying an end of their sign taking the opportunity to let onlookers know the group existed. No one was following. The groups were comprised mostly of women dressed in what looked like their Sunday-go-to-meeting clothes, they seemed genuinely pleased just to be participating in the parade.

Bringing up the rear like comic relief was a small work crew of men dressed in old trousers complete with hammers and other tools hanging from their work belts having a good ol' time waving and smiling at their friends. Their banner read—*For Wood Stove Installation and Home Repair call Manny at...*

Next came an equestrian group. Horses decked out in polished and buffed saddles and harnesses adorned with silver, turquoise and malachite fittings were ridden by Navajo men wearing large turquoise rings and bola ties. Some of them had long braids coming out from under their cowboy hats that could be seen only when they passed. Brand new rope wound in neat circles and looped around saddle horns, was hanging against the recently curried animals, added to the parade's festive spirit. Every one of them was sitting tall in the saddle, not looking around as if they were leading the way for something grand. These riders were dressed up in long sleeves shirts and new jeans and polished cowboy boots. They played to the crowd by keeping their animals as controlled as they were along the way. In a western town such as Gallup, equestrian talent and horsemanship are greatly appreciated and I could tell by the cheering they were a crowd favorite.

The spectators were just as interesting to watch as the parade, almost more so. Standing along the street were grandmothers as remnants of the distant past, some with scarves wrapped under their necks, others showing hair buns knotted at the back of their heads elegantly set with silver combs, watching patiently with their families. Everyone seemed to know everyone else, and on the whole the crowd was subdued and reserved. I didn't hear one wise-crack or one boisterous remark during the entire parade.

Then I saw why. Slowly the people watching stood as a small group of hoary-headed Navajo men came into view. All talking subsided as the men solemnly walked by and was replaced by a gradual and building applause; it was a dramatic moment as the remaining Navajo Code Talkers proudly moved through with little fanfare other than our growing applause. Wearing light yellow shirts decorated with war emblems of honor and soft brimless rust colored hats and black dress shoes they walked with all the nobility of crown princes with dignity, pride and honor, holding their heads up high for the vital contribution they made during W.W.II in Guadalcanal, Iwo Jima, and Okinawa by devising a code using their native tongue. Serving in the South Pacific as marines, they used their complex Navajo language, which uses four separate tones of voice—low, high, rising and falling, that proved to be impossible for the Japanese to crack.[12]

Watching Franklin from across the street clapping enthusiastically, I knew this was the reason he wanted me to see the parade, because when the code talkers left their mark on the world, he must have felt it was his mark as well. I suppose patriotism was all Franklin had left.

The parade made me happy: the sky stayed friendly and I'd learned some remarkable Navaho history. I walked back to the car filled with an indebtedness for the contribution the brave Code Talkers made. Walking alongside Franklin, I had a new respect for him, a true patriot.

Chapter 15—Off the Beaten Trail

The best thing about working at St. Francis Retreat was, it didn't feel like work. In the wide open spaces there was no one looking over my shoulder questioning my every decision, the only harassing presence was the continual heavy silence pressing on my ears like a one-note flute. This could be intimidating but to me I felt privileged to listen to the awesome sound 'quiet' makes on its own.

It was mid-week with no retreats on and I was cleaning the large retreat bell in the middle of the front yard. Bushy brown squirrels were scampering about in quick light runs, red headed woodpeckers were stroking repeatedly at dried trunks of trees, and birds were stretching their vocals chords in miniature arias.

As I fingered the bell's heavy clapper, I thought how sounds had the ability to affect my moods; the gentle clinking of a chain against a pole could put me in a mesmeric stupor, listening to leaves shivering their way from branch to branch stirred nostalgic longings, a peal of bells turned the present into bitter-sweet longings of former times lost through the years. But there are few sounds more evocative than a car moving in the distance. It is a forlorn, almost hopeless sound and I loved hearing it. Often at night I lay listening to trains as they moved through Gallup. The entrancing change in pitch was haunting and left me lonely. I pictured the driver alone too, two souls alone in the night.

Continuing to clean the bell, I guided the clapper to its side, but let it go when I heard a car traveling on the highway in front of the retreat center. Listening for the Doppler[13] change in pitch I was surprised when it didn't happen. Instead, the fast moving car had slowed and was moving up our driveway. With the sound of rubber treading on gravel getting closer and closer, in a short skid the vehicle stopped. And breaking the silence like a rude awakening, I heard the familiar loud voice of Sr. Carol call, "Yay te hey, Anne!"

Waiting for the dust to settle around her dirty Bronco, I approached the creaking vehicle as it rested in a sifting cloud of dust. Steeling myself and making sure my feet were flat on the ground, I answered back, "Howdy!"

She was our nearest neighbor, missionary Sr. Carol, Bible thumping, Scripture quoting, Amen ending, evangelical Sister Carol dedicated to converting heathens, and who I suspected had me at the top of her list. This one-woman envoy set out with good works, sacraments, and Gospel teachings to carry out appointed salvations by faith. Trips to the reservation were worth the preaching even though she went about saving my soul with all the zeal of an encyclopedia salesman. For this reason, my mind blew a trumpet blast whenever she drove in to herald her entrance.

I could have told her I'd tried to become a nun and had actually been in a novitiate so we were fighting the same good fight and that I knew all about the *slippery slope*, but my experience with eager religious, is that nothing I could have said would ever change her opinion of me; I would always be a God-forsaken little waif who needed the simplest passages explained. Which might me true, I am not very adept at quoting Scripture other than knowing if a passage came from the Old Testament or the New. Abiding by them is the important thing.

With the encouragement of Sr. Hyacinth to experience as much as I could, I hopped in and we pulled the car doors closed behind us and took off. It was always adventurous going on the reservation, I thought, almost like daring something to happen. The hogans were set acres apart on fields covered with old dry scrub bushes and weeds. There were no trees and no lawns understandably, since the reservation doesn't have running water; it was one gigantic flat field. I didn't see any businesses so I understood why Sr. Carol needed to deliver supplies to a family who had lost the support of their bread winner, Robert, after he had been kicked in the ribs by a mule.

In driving, Sr. Carol used three gears: forward, full steam ahead, and get out the way. Without hesitating she turned this way and that until I was totally lost. I had to marvel again at her keen sense of direction on these intersecting dirt roads winding through fields and hogans. Every place looked the same. The only difference I could see in the octagonal hogans (especially since each one faced in the same direction, east) was that a few roofs had vegetables growing out of them; tomatoes, onions, garlic.

Miles in, I noticed we hadn't passed any gas stations in case we had car trouble or had to ask for directions. Sr. Carol followed an unwavering course that had no signs marking streets, no name-plates identifying families, and this I was sure Sister appreciated, no speed limits posted. I didn't think she would have stopped to ask for directions anyway because after all the years she had been saving lost souls here, I didn't think she would ever admit to being lost herself.

We didn't have one moment of daring as we juddered and shook along the dirt roads to our destination. Sr. Carol knew where she was going and how to get there so I pushed aside any misgivings and went along for the ride. I had to trust her driving ability but there was nothing to worry about here, she was a skilled driver. In the days before mandatory seat belts, the hard part was staying in my seat. I held onto or braced myself against the top of the dash board, under the dash, the ashtray, underneath my seat, the roof, or on the edges of my open window.

While her physical eyes were riveted on the road, her inner eyes concentrated on my soul as she said, "How straight is the gate and how narrow the way that leadeth unto eternal life!" To my astonishment however, I noticed the more filled with religious fervor she became, the more she pushed on the accelerator. When she finished with, "There are few that find it!" the tires suddenly caught after sliding around a corner and we almost flew headfirst into life everlasting there and then. As the car straightened, I vowed to do better in life.

The front door was wide open on the hogan when we pulled up, meaning it had been taken completely off. I stayed in the car while Sister approached the hogan. Although it was dim inside I could see beds lining the far wall and a wood stove in the center with a gray metal pail on top of it. The hogan looked cramped and I was glad I decided to stay behind, especially after seeing a lizard scurrying out making for the light.

With Robert's wife Helena helping, the three of us carried cardboard boxes full of supplies containing corn, rice and beans, flour, sugar, red and green chilies, sunflower seeds among other food items to the entry where we left them neatly stacked near the front door.

Helena thanked us and politely waited until we drove off the property before turning and walking back inside the dark hogan. I looked at Sr. Carol and watched as she readied herself for the drive home. She straightened the rear view mirror, reached around to the window to flick a bug from her field of vision, adjusted the position of her seat before finally turning the key. Gunning the engine it wouldn't have surprised me to see her pull out a pair of leather gloves from under the seat for the drive home.

We left with the knowledge we had helped a family in need; waves of benevolence poured from our conversation as we wished them well then went on our way. I looked back at the hogan and saw smoke rising from a rusty pipe sticking out of a hole in the roof and it gave me a good feeling inside to think maybe the whispy condensation of color, smoke, smell and ash over the hogan was from the foodstuff we'd left.

"Good driving, Sister," I encouraged, hoping she'd take my meaning to heart. But as our car bottomed out over a shoulder I knew my left-handed compliment had been taken seriously.

The ride seemed shorter on the way back with no expectations to look forward to. I was glad to see the turnoff to the Retreat Center but my relief was short-lived as we drove within yards of the drive.

"What's that?" I wondered, pointing to a straw figure at the base of the drive.

"Looks like someone was upset," Carol answered, suddenly brisk. "It's a dummy of a person and the edges have been singed, otherwise known as a figure burned in effigy. It happens out here, not frequently, but it happens."

We pulled alongside, slowed, but didn't get out. I could tell Sr. Carol wasn't in a hurry to investigate and she pulled away and continued our ascent. I had the feeling she didn't want to be seen anywhere its vicinity.

A growing sense of foreboding crept over me by the time we reached the statue of Jesus at the top of the hill and when Carol said, "Make sure you tell Hyacinth about this," I knew it wasn't a good sign.

Standing outside the Bronco, it felt good to close the door and walk on steady ground and let the peacefulness of the retreat grounds invade my spirit. I watched as Sr. Carol once again pounced on the accelerator sending the car lurching forward on the way to her parish. Maybe the model name on the car had something to do with it but there was a moment as I watched her move the car away the impression came to me of Sister flapping a cowboy hat against the side of the vehicle to make it go faster.

I heard her call out one last spiritual epithet as she rode off into the sunset. I'm sure it must have been "Hallelujah," but it sounded an awful lot like, "Ye ha!"

I assumed Doppler's principle must have affected my hearing, so I gave her the benefit of the doubt.

Chapter 16—An Effigy

My mind was working as I walked to the porch in front of the retreat trying to remember what I knew, if anything, about figures in effigy. One picture came to mind of a man sneaking into a cellar to hide a stash of gunpowder. It was the only incident I could recall having anything to do with an 'effigy' and I dredged it up it from my high school history class text book. It came back to me through a little black and white drawing, a sketch of a man cowering by himself in a cellar. The more I walked, the clearer the image became.

Sr. Hyacinth was sitting at the table in the small dining room stirring sugar in her cup of coffee when I walked in. "You must be hungry after your trip to the reservation," she said. "I've never known Sr. Carol to stop for a meal on the road, with her it's always go, go, go. That's probably why she's so skinny," pushing an empty plate toward me while she tried to unravel the enigma of Carol's weight maintenance.

"You're right there, we didn't stop to eat anywhere, I agreed. "But then again I didn't see one fast food place along the way either. For that matter, I only remember passing one other vehicle on the way, there and back, so there wouldn't be much drive-through business."

Tapping her spoon against the side of her cup, she turned to me and asked, "How was it? Did you see anything interesting?"

"As a matter of fact, we did see something of interest, but it wasn't on the reservation, it was at the base of our driveway."

"What?" Hyacinth asked.

"That's right. Someone dropped off a straw dummy right at our entrance. Sr. Carol thought it was a figure burned in effigy because it had been singed around the edges," I explained.

"What?" she asked again, almost shouting, a wide-eyed look replacing her usual jovial manner.

"No kidding. An entire body: head, arms, and legs, feet and hands.

Quite disturbing actually. Wire is holding the thing together," trying to be as calm as I could.

"Are you sure? Could Sr. Carol have been mistaken?"

"No. You can't mistake a thing like this."

"Well, it can't stay there," she barked in finality. "Tomorrow morning we'll to go to the group home and bring the truck back so we can throw the thing in the back and get it out of here."

I was trembling a little as we discussed why someone would do such a thing, but nothing ever seemed to disturb Sr. Hyacinth. She worked it through logically, we weren't the only people living on this road. Nothing ever got her down, noticing how soon a smile was back on her face as she walked to the kitchen to serve me dinner from food warming on the stove.

That night I had a strange dream. I was walking in an underground room in between tubs held together with wooden hoops. A free swinging light bulb illumined cobwebs at the end of an aisle as I searched for a way out. The place was dark and shadowy and I could feel a chilling cold like the hand of death. There was a constant sound of a discussion taking place in the background although I couldn't see any faces. At times loud noises made me look harder for the way out, but when I realized the doors were without handles and I was trapped, I woke up with a jolt.

Early the next day, both of us were eager to inspect the straw figure, Sr. Hyacinth drove us to collect the truck from the girl's home. On the way down we saw it was still propped up against the side of our hill on the edge of our drive, nobody had touched it during the night. Just knowing the responsible party wasn't wandering around last night doing mischief was a relief in itself, and we raced into Gallup to the girl's home on this little wave of optimism.

"I spoke with Sr. Celeste last night, she knows what's going on," Hyacinth said, as she jumped in, threw it in gear and we shot back to the retreat center.

She pulled in as close as she could to the bulky figure and we hopped out. The ominous part of whole thing was not what it looked like, as hideous as it was, but the fact that someone had gone to all the trouble to make it and drag it close to the retreat in the dead of night. It was unsettling to know a very angry person was among our acquaintances. It made me wonder if retreat directors working in urban areas had to contend with rural practices such as this.

We tried to avoid touching the burnt ends. With Sister taking the head and me grabbing the calves, we swung somebody's indignation in the back of the truck and drove to the retreat where we pulled the pieces of the dry cut straw apart.

Remnants of the dream I had the night before stayed with me in feelings and I was able to fit more of the pieces of my memory together. Over breakfast I told Sister about what I could recall about burning in effigy, that what stood out most in my mind was a Gunpowder Plot I had read about in a history class. I didn't remember the plot, per se, I remembered a little black and white sketch of a man cowering in a cellar is what stood out in my mind.

That man was Guy Fawkes, a conspirator who was in charge of filling barrels of gunpowder in the cellar to blow up the House of Lords in England.[14] Four other conspirators, including Fawkes, were rounded up, tried, and executed for treason. "And to this day," I told Hyacinth, "The United Kingdom acknowledges his actions by burning him in effigy."

"That doesn't make me feel any better!" she said with a smile and a raised eyebrow.

We never had a mention from any retreatants and we considered the straw dummy must have been meant for somewhere else up the road. I think Hyacinth was as unnerved about the assemblage of intimidation as I was though. We startled easily, and once unaware I was coming out of the dining room when she was going in, we both nearly jumped out of our skins.

The incident was hard to shake and made me look over my shoulder more for about a week thereafter before it eventually slipped out of mind and was forgotten. Not entirely though when I thought about it. As I went to sleep, I did thank God hogans weren't built with wine cellars.

Chapter 17—The Compleat Jesuit

Under the window in the back of the tan sedan I noticed a felt hat like the kind fishermen wear as the car coasted by me through the retreat yard. My curiosity now set, I waited until I heard the emergency brake tread down and a car door slam, and the sound of footsteps walking away before stepping into the visible track of dust left in its wake. When I was convinced the car was totally stopped, I inched toward it treating it like it was some wayward creature that had washed in with so much waif or estray cast into our yard. The closer I came, the more I began to feel a red tide spreading across my face displaying the very action I was trying to conceal: snooping. Being caught red-handed would not be a good first impression.

But were those really ordinary garment buttons I saw pinned all over the felt hat? Or were they floating decoys designed to entice denizens of the deep? I hoped the colorful headdress wasn't used in a passing the hat portion of a traveling show, and disguised my approach to the back of the car by taking calcuiated giant steps over the partially completed rock paths like a stone skipping over a lake top.

Gripped between wanting to know what was pinned to that hat and my conscience telling me to stop tugging on the driver's fishing line, I found myself wading knee deep in curiosity.

So, keeping a watchful eye on the office door in case it should suddenly open, I slunk closer, moving in and away, each time becoming a little braver and a little closer. Fearful of being found out, I looked around again for witnesses making sure the coast was clear, then went forward comfortable in the audible hush of quiet with the engine turned off.

I pulled up to the car to hurriedly inspect my catch before my nerves got the better of me and I would be compelled to release it from sight. Beginning in the front seat, I nonchalantly looked in and saw a small red ice chest in the center of the bench seat. This made me happy for what self-respecting fisherman would be caught in the middle of a lake without sandwiches and drinks? It was a good sign. Next to the ice chest was a wad of clothes that had been tossed in without regard to the crumpled look. Another good sign; spending all day in a boat cutting bait and untangling lines was messy business and indicated a certain amount of indifference to his appearance; the owner of this car was not about to hold out his pinkie whenever he sipped his favorite tea.

What I saw resting on the back shelf made me do a double-take. Lying on the ledge was a purple hat all right, but what I hadn't seen when the car rolled through the yard were lures, *not* buttons, made from bunches of feathers of different colors: orange with black stripes, purple with blue stripes, green with black stripes, all brandishing shiny barbed hooks. As I looked fixedly at the hat, I noticed one lure sporting two hooks set back to back, making it look like an anchor. It was full of thick bristles of orange feathers camouflaging dark hooks. I knew this had to be his favorite lure guaranteed to entice the most reluctant cold-blooded fish to bite.

I felt a wave of panic after hearing clicking sounds coming from the office doorknob and decided to turn and walk directly toward the opening door to meet whoever was coming out head on. This would show whoever I met I wasn't up to anything and had nothing to hide.

"This is Fr. Lighterman," Sr. Hyacinth introduced, "our new resident chaplain. The bishop stationed him here after Father spent two years acting as chaplain in a school for Indians on the outskirts of Gallup. I guess there's a certain progression here, retreatants are students too, only they learn about God."

I was used to Hyacinth springing surprises on me by this time. But with a name like Lighterman and owner of a fisherman's hat, I expected to meet, in keeping with his name, a diminutive, lithe, and fit figure of a man; a real sportsman. Was I surprised when he stepped around out in front of Hyacinth! I had never seen a belly this size on a person before, man or woman! Thinking about it, it came to me that fishing was the perfect mesh between man and sport; what other sport could he spend hours reeling in a meal while thinking about which recipe to try and feeling his mouth water every time a fish jumped? With his inordinate enjoyment of food I thought fishing was just the sport for him, it was a natural.

"Father will be saying daily Mass for us in the chapel. We haven't decided on the time yet, I'll let you know, and he's welcome to join us for Office recital as well," Hyacinth mentioned as the three of us walked to the chapel. (More often than not, when the retreat schedule didn't conflict, I joined the three sisters reciting the Office, evening out the back and forth recitation of the psalms with two people on each side.) Walking behind them, I saw Father Lighterman was a couple inches shorter than Hyacinth, and seeing the sparse strands of silver hair on the back of his neck, he was older too.

I was introduced to Father and was grateful Sr. Hyacinth didn't mention I had MS. Maybe she'd forgotten because I was so physically adept and my body acted completely normal. When he clasped my hand in greeting I wondered if our new chaplain would offer to help Franklin spread rocks over the paths, but by the feel of his soft pudgy hand, I didn't think he would. I turned out to be right. I guess it's better to have a prayerful preacher whose hands were soft from turning pages of his Bible anyway.

"We'll put you in one of the front bedrooms on the side of the chapel," Hyacinth directed, "it has a nice warm feel to it," opening the door so he could see the orange drapes hanging above the apricot colored rug. "This is a new building and right now there isn't anybody else here, so you'll have the whole building to yourself. This might change of course, when we have a large retreat and the hogans are full, but I'll hold off the overflow as long as I can. Tomorrow I'll give you the grand tour, but right now, let's get your car unpacked," prompting us into action by a directional nod of her head. "You can pull up close to the hallway door," pointing out there was proper outside lighting at the entrance.

We walked back over to his car with him and waited as he opened the passenger door. Finally I could ask about the hat and find out how much of a fisherman he really was. He scooped up the clothes off the front seat and handed some shirts to me. Since most of the short sleeved shirts were white, I was struck by a red bandanna tucked in and partly showing sticking out from one of the pockets. But with white polka dots?

I walked to his room and dropped the shirts on one of the two twin beds while he backed the car in as close as he could to the door. The kerchief stood out like a red chili pepper against the white shirts and the orange bedspread, and Sr. Hyacinth and I smiled at each other at his taste in fashion. Priest or not, this was a one weird fashion statement.

Waiting for an opening in the conversation to work in lake shores and riverbeds, the subject was brought up for me the moment he unlocked the trunk. In all seriousness, he turned to face us and said, "This is where I store my gentleness of mind and serenity of spirit. Good man, that Washington Irving." And lifting the trunk wide open, I saw a jumble of poles and collapsible rods, nets and pliers, fishing boxes, and a couple deteriorating knives that looked like they had seen more than their share of fish gutting. "I never get my line wet without wearing my lucky handkerchief," pointing to the bold kerchief, making Sr. Hyacinth and I to smile at each other. He was a serious fisherman all right!

"I *may* have seen it. Is it red?" trying not to show interest in prying into his personal effects.

He looked pleased I had asked. A faraway look, followed by a physical calm came over his face as he must have thought about all the times his special handkerchief had helped him reel in the big one. "The stories I could tell you!"

"Oh, but Father. I have the story to end all stories," I assured him, "and if I hadn't seen it with my eyes, I *never* would have believed it," I countered.

"If you two are going to start swapping tales about the one that got away, let's do it over coffee and cake," Sr. Hyacinth said, "but after we get the car unloaded."

The three of us made short work of settling Father in his new quarters, prompted by the thought of cake and hot coffee waiting for us. As I watched Sr. Hyacinth pour the coffee, I told myself to be as reserved as I could, because as unbelievable as my story was, I didn't want Fr. Lighterman's first impression of me to be a brazen-faced boaster, even though I knew I had the fishing story to end all fishing stories.

I don't know if Father's mood was cheered considerably at the prospect of having an audience willing to listen to his past fishing exploits, or at the fact that we were about to eat homemade chocolate cake, but he wasted no time in narrating particular times portraying his luck and endurance the sport requires. He described in detail the weight, length and color of each sizable catch, how long it took each one to land, and what type of bait he used for each fish, culminating with the inevitable "one that got away" story in every fisherman's repertoire. For his *coup de grâce*, he brought out his lucky hat. Handling it with kid gloves because of the hooks, he displayed it by placing his fist under the crown and gingerly turned it around giving us a view of every one of his colorful lures, showing us what it's like to be crowned with success.

His stories were all well and good, but very predictable, even for a priest who made a living thinking up interesting homilies to keep churchgoers in their seats. Around his third fish, I began picturing him in each accounting, as a bear-like figure wearing the faded purple hat, in his red handkerchief with white polka dots knotted around his neck, holding a cane pole wedged in tightly beside his stomach as he snagged an open can of discarded pork and beans with his two sided lure, happy to have caught *something* as he sat contentedly in the grass among white daisies and purple lilacs watching the water drip, drip, drip as he lifted the dented can out of the water with his pole. "More cake anybody?" jolted me back.

We shifted to more comfortable positions in our chairs while Sr. Hyacinth warmed our coffee with refills. "More cake anybody?" she offered again as she dropped a slice on each of our plates without waiting to hear our answers.

"Don't mind if I do. How can *talking* give me such an appetite?" Fr. Lighterman pondered with out loud, acting mystified by the silliness of it.

From this first meeting, he seemed humble, likable and mild-mannered, as most people usually are who aspire to be as poor in spirit as Christ. But it was when he asked, "Have you ever heard of better stories than these?" that I felt genuinely sorry I had to upstage him.

"As a matter of fact, Father, have I got a story about the one that got away."

"Just a minute, it only counts if you took the hook out of its mouth," he said pointedly followed by half a smile, like he was an authority from the *Fish & Game Department.*

I pushed back from the table a little like I needed plenty of room to tell my story, and hoped Father didn't think it was for my embellishments.

Growing up by the ocean along with brothers and a father who liked to fish, I naturally learned too. My sisters and I had our share of finding fish scales in our hair from deck hands scattering bait over the water as they chummed, as I thought back to the many excursions we took on half-day boats.

One summer, I drove with my brother Ed, who prided himself on being a good fisherman, to Oregon after reading how good the fishing was at a particular lake. It sounded like fun, so on hot summer's day we started out. And of course, Ed had his lucky fishing pole in the back of the truck.

During the drive whenever he'd talk about landing 'the big one,' which was quite often, out of habit I would end his thought with the harmless, "God willing," just to help our chances.

At one point he turned to me and said adamantly, "God has nothing to do with whether I catch a big fish or not, it's skill."

Arriving at the lake we stopped in at the rustic store for bait & tackle and bought a container of worms, but not any worms, these were Oregon worms, and they were they were all big, fat, and juicy. He would poke around in the stuffed container of dirt trying to find the littlest big one he could for me so I could bait my own hook. The longer we trolled in the row boat using worm after worm, there came a point when there weren't any little ones left wiggling in the confused jumble.

Motorboats were prohibited so we rowed around the quiet lake by paddling oars for about an hour, taking in the fluffy white clouds, the pointed hill tops surrounding us in forests of green, and birds of prey circling over us in noiseless glides. Having only a few bites, we decided to pull up on land and fish from shore.

Casting out, Ed secured his pole at the end of our grounded row boat before walking over to me to bait my hook. While he fiddled baiting my hook with the biggest worm I have ever seen, that's when we heard the splash. We looked at each other aghast, stricken with the shock of knowing what that splash was; the sound of Ed's lucky pole going into the drink. In a flash, he threw down the worms and we ran up and over the embankment to have our worst fear confirmed, there was no pole at the end of the rowboat. "There goes my lucky pole!" he said, dejectedly.

I couldn't bring myself to say anything. What could I possibly say to someone who was doing me the favor by baiting my hook, and it cost him his rig? We stood silently looking only at the ripples caused by the sinking spool. There was nothing left, no bait, no reel, no pole. It was all gone. His lucky pole had gone to a watery grave, done in by a large Oregon fish.

We were still standing on the bank in shock when suddenly a huge fish jumped out of the water in the center of the lake which made me feel worse, Ed could have had a fish like that if I hadn't asked him to bait my hook…when suddenly, a big fish jumped again, then again, almost in the same spot. "That's my fish!" shouted Ed. Then the lake went quiet."That's my fish. I know it was!" Then out of the blue we heard another splash, this time coming from a different location, and it too, began jumping in one spot. A beautiful rainbow trout.

Running back over the embankment towards the new splash site, putting two and two together, my brother figured the fish was dragging his pole around the lake while it was trying to free itself and the pole kept getting caught, forcing the fish to jump.

"I'm going in!" Ed yelled, ripping off his tennis shoes.

"You're joking!" I yelled back. You know how icy lake water is? And besides, you said these are cutthroat trout. They have teeth!"

"I know," he shivered, already standing up to his knees in the lake.

Without hesitation, he let himself sink into the freezing water, popping up suddenly, gasping for air from the first shock. Plunging in again, he swam farther out, and again came up for air. I watched him do this repeatedly but about the fifth try, he popped out of the water yelling, "I see it! I can see it! My pole's caught on a big log!" With no time to think, he took a big gulp of air and dove to the pole and freed it, bursting out of the water holding it above his head up like a trophy. Once his bare feet found stable footing on the jagged rocks and stones on the bank, he began reeling.

"What are you doing that for?" I asked.

"The fish is still on the line!" he yelled back excitedly.

"It still has the hook in it mouth?" I yelled, unable to believe after all this time the fish hadn't dislodged it.

"Yeah, but it's exhausted from dragging the pole around the lake and doesn't have much fight left," Andy screamed back. "I'll have to play it as gently as I can and try not to jerk out the hook."

"You can try," I said, "but as fast as the fish was running I hope it doesn't try to swim back out to the middle of the lake again."

"It's too tired," he said. "Here, take the pole."

"What for?" I asked, surprised.

"I think I can grab the line and *pull* it in!"

I watched dumbfounded as Ed felt along the line which was invisible in the water except for the metal ring on the eyelet and followed the line out as far as he could and literally pulled the huge fish safely up on shore. As we stood there watching the beautiful blue, green and gold fish flopping in the dirt, we looked at each other and started to laugh, not at the doomed fish, it was more from hysterical relief at the best outcome we could have imagined: at Ed's intrepid actions, at his safe return, at not getting tangled up in debris from a wrecked boat or being caught on a log, and best of all, at retrieving his lucky pole.

"Not many people would dive into freezing water after a fish!" I kidded.

"I know! The worst part was not knowing what was down there. I could have seen anything down there, rusted car frames, skeletons, Oregon leeches for all I know!" he said, laughing in relief.

"Yeah, I was worried you'd get tangled up on some branch and couldn't come up. I wasn't about to dive in after you!" We both laughed. In fact we couldn't stop laughing, the entire incident was just so bizarre. Words couldn't convey the strangeness of what we were feeling. Now, during the remainder of the trip every time we looked at each other, we would shake our heads in disbelief and say over and over, "I *don't* believe it!"

I brought out my camera and snapped numerous pictures for the record of Ed in his trunks, dripping wet, proudly holding the colorful trout to show it from various angles: laying it on the ground, holding it over his head, next to a beer for prospective, and one or two close ups of its big mouth (the fish's, that is).

Back at the bait shop, we felt very distinguished to find out Ed's fish weighed a whopping 14 1/2 lbs. and was the largest trout ever pulled from the lake! Admirers crowded around but we didn't mention *how* it was caught, only that it was one that *didn't* get away. Ed shared his good fortune by dividing the fillets with a couple of mountain men who looked like they could use a good meal, while I tacked up one of the pictures of Ed holding his record trout along with its specs on the back of the door with all the other pictures of anglers and fish, that is probably still there today.

Later, when we were on our way home, Ed said in uncharacteristic seriousness, "I will never doubt I had a worm on one end and God on the other."

"No doubt in my mind at all either."

"Look, we have only have 300 miles to go," he said, pointing at the sign on the freeway. "God willing."

Sr. Hyacinth didn't know what to make of my fishing story, whether to believe it or not, I could tell by her vague comment she offered, "Thanks for sharing it anyway," she said, as she began taking our plates and cups into the kitchen. Not being an angler, I realized, she couldn't fully appreciate any fishing story.

It was impossible to tell what Fr. Lighterman thought about it, simply saying, "Good story, good story," as he got up from the table. I was hoping for something more personal like, *"That's some fishing story!"* From his rather lackluster assessment and analysis, I couldn't tell what he *really* thought. Until…

It was time for Father's first Mass in the retreat chapel the next day. There were no retreatants so we were a small group, three Franciscan nuns and myself. Everything was going along fine; the holy water founts were filled, the pages were marked for the readings, the key to the tabernacle was in place.

Out of all the topics Father could have picked to use as his homily, he chose a story about a Spanish senorita in the seventeenth century who had been caught committing adultery. For her punishment she was to be publicly stoned in the town's bull ring. As she was being pummeled with rocks, with her final breath she had the wherewithal to reach down and cover her legs with her skirt, right before she died.

One would think the sermon Father delivered would pertain to the subject at hand. His homiletic preaching at least mentioning modesty, citing immorality, specifying the harmful effects of adultery, maybe expounding the power that comes from virtuous behavior perhaps glossing over the cardinal virtues.[15] Instead, for the next ten minutes Father lectured on dishonesty, untruthfulness, mendacity and deception.

I never was for sure if his homily was directed at me or was just an uncomfortable coincidence, but in my heart I finally knew what he thought of my fishing story.

Chapter 18—Fear and Loathing

Being frightened is no fun. The fact that Sr. Hyacinth was staying in another building a half an acre away didn't help matters, I was still living by myself in a hogan without a phone and had to deal with every creak, bump, and suspicious noise I heard on my own. There was no doubt about it, my sleeping had become a whole lot sounder ever since I knew she was back.

The first night I spent in the hogan wasn't too unnerving because I was too tired from traveling and from the emotional drain of meeting the prospective director to be scared. As tired as I was, before I went to bed, I made myself go through each bedroom and check the sliding glass doors to make sure they were locked, forced myself to look under each bed for hidden predators, and open every closet searching for would-be abductors and nefarious ne'er-do-wells. Maybe the sight of me walking through the hogan holding a hefty pine branch filled with jagged knotholes would make an intruder have second thoughts. I placed this branch next to my bed every night…just in case.

I have always been a light sleeper and this nightly ritual gave me a sense of confidence I was absolutely alone and my quarters were secure. Only then, would I allow myself to drop off to sleep. It wasn't until Hyacinth suddenly had to go to Tucson for her brother's funeral that I began putting a desk chair behind the front door to alert me to an intruder. There was nothing worth stealing in the hogan anyway, except my person, and I didn't know how much respect a burglar would show this kind of church property. Probably none.

Fear moves through my mind with lightning speed if I'd let it. If each unidentifiable noise is not discovered and its source discounted immediately by reason, fear will disturb my sense of well-being and make my imagination sit bolt upright. I made a point never to watch movies that would frighten me out of my wits, and I especially avoided watching graphic movies that could make my flesh crawl or were marked with unusual amounts of gore, bloodshed or violence. Possession movies in which the mind loses its balance I avoided altogether, I had had enough anxiety in my life. I did this purposely so I could maintain my composure for situations I was in now; I did not want to be on my own somewhere and have scenes of homicidal butchers running through my mind from some movie I'd seen years before. If I was going to come to an untimely end, I wanted it to be unrehearsed.

The second night in my hogan did not go as smoothly as the first. Invigorated by the previous night's sleep caused by exhaustion, I lay in bed with my arms under the blankets and the covers pulled up to eyes. I looked like I was ready for sleep; teeth were brushed and my pajamas were on, the lights were off, and my eyes were closed. But thirty minutes of useless trying told me differently, bringing anxious thoughts of being at the retreat center with no one within shouting distance. As a last resort: *Oh, Angel of God, my guardian dear to whom God's love entrusts me here. Ever this day be at my side to light, to guard, to rule, and guide. Amen.* Its powerful lilt couldn't hurt.

I started thinking of the most frightening night I'd ever spent. I had gone camping with my family and to make it more adventurous, together with my younger brothers and sister and a teenage friend, Jeff, we pleaded to have our tent pitched up on a small hill away from parental earshot. This was a big mistake, for out of a sound sleep I was awakened by the sound of footsteps that started at the bottom of the hill and continued to the outside of our large tent. Out of a sound sleep at first, I became wide awake very quickly following the sound of the slow walking boots until they came to a stop, right behind my head not a foot away!

Aware that the only thing between me and this stranger was a thin piece of canvas that could easily be sliced open with a hunting knife, the rest of the night I hardly breathed, let alone move. I slept as stiff and straight as a steel rod, and in no time I was covered in a hot sweat that drenched my whole body, but I wasn't about to call attention to myself by stretching. Besides, I had the others in the tent to think of as well.

I stayed awake the entire night listening for the calculating prowler on the outside of the tent to make his move. I wanted to be ready. Needless to say, I said my guardian angel prayer with deep conviction many times that night.

I was never so glad to see the dawn come as that morning, or have someone else wake up! I remember whispering to our friend, "Jeff, there's someone standing right behind me outside the tent. I heard him walk up last night and he never went away."

I'll never forget the speed in which he unzipped his sleeping bag and kicked his way free and unzipped the tent flap, and with little regard to his own personal safety, strode to the back of the tent. In two seconds, he stuck his head back inside the tent and announced his findings, "There's no one out there," he said relieved. With the disturbed look of 'you must be crazy,' he crawled back into the warmth of his sleeping bag.

"That can't be," I insisted, still sotto voce. "I heard someone walk up just as clearly as I'm talking to you now, and he didn't walk away!"

"Go look for yourself," not mad at all by my throwing a scare into his morning. Judging from the amount of fear which he heard in my strained voice, he could tell I was deadly serious.

Allowing myself to stretch for the first time that night, I struggled out my sleeping bag unzipping the long zipper, and climbed out of the tent. Careful not to disturb any footprints I saw, I walked around to the back of the tent and very carefully searched the surrounding dirt. How could this be? There wasn't one print of a boot or shoe print anywhere in the dirt where I figured they should be, right up close to the canvas. I couldn't believe it, and worse yet, I realized this night of physical and mental torment was of my own making! Every painful leg cramp, crick, kink, and warm drip of perspiration that rolled down my face I had done to myself had been for nothing.

Tucked in my bed in my hogan thinking back on that night, I tried to understand what happened, and why my imagination created the whole frightening escapade. Was it showing me my worst fear? A stranger coming out of nowhere and waiting to pounce at the right moment? It truly was the most scared I've ever been in my life and for such a prolonged period. Not wanting to bring on a reenactment by thinking about it, I decided I would never know, and forced myself to think of happier, cheerful moments. Like the time I dressed up for Halloween in the monastery.

Fear has a place in bringing a person closer to God. Some Retreat Centers offer the seclusion of hermitages for people who want to voluntarily welcome this feeling of exile. A slight state of dread with no one to call on but God may easily unite a frightened person to the All Powerful Rescuer very quickly.

I was doubly grateful I had the foresight years ago not to fill my mind with realistic, terrifying scenes from movies. I did all right creating them on my own.

Chapter 19—A Benny and Joon Diaconate

As I pushed back the golden folds of the drapes in the new retreat building and pulled open the window to air the room, I began to think that springing surprises on Sr. Hyacinth was the bishop's modus operandi instead of a lack of preparedness. Getting the drop on people by taking them unawares avoided possible defensive stands and counter oppositions to why the undertaking shouldn't take place, like stationing Fr. Lighterman here as chaplain with little or no forewarning. This time the surprises were named Walter and June and they were here for the summer.

A deacon is a cleric who ranks below priests in the Anglican, Eastern Orthodox and Roman Catholic churches, or a Protestant lay person who assists the minister. I had never worked with any of this kind of deaconry before but with their arrival I was about to learn an incontestable truth from Sr. Hyacinth; the bishop can do anything he wants.

"They'll be a great help to the retreat the bishop assured me," Sr. Hyacinth coerced, trying to get me to come round to her resigned attitude. "After all, what if something should happen to Franklin? Then where would we be?"

"We can use the help all right," I'd reassured her, trusting deacon Walter would have some practical maintenance experience or at least know which side of the hammer to hold.

"Bishop Struther wasn't hesitant in voicing their praises either," Hyacinth assured. "June, the deacon's wife will keep her hands out of her pockets too, the bishop said she'll work right along her husband, and the fact they are his personal friends shouldn't sway our judgment about assigning them work," prompting my eyes to wander over the grounds looking for work for them.

I watched as a black shiny car pulled up to the office and knew a car without any of Gallup's road mud splattered on its sides had to be carrying someone important, and wondered if Fr. Lighterman at the other side of the retreat building had noticed it too; top-ranking people always drew attention by their prominence, as if importance is somehow superimposed on another by proximity alone.

Through the curtains I could make out a middle aged woman struggling out of the front seat, stretch, and reach back in the car for her purse. A middle aged man followed her. Next I watched as the driver got out and opened the passenger door while a tall man wearing black dress slacks and jacket stepped from the car's back seat. Good heavens, is that the bishop? Minus the miter? It is!

I watched as the driver quickly went to the suited gentleman's side to await orders in a docile display of fetch and carry. He unloaded the trunk of the car while the suited man looked on and stood quietly at the Bishop's side. Alerted by the commotion, moments later Sr. Hyacinth appeared from the office. I could hear her welcoming each one with a warm yah-te-hey greeting, reminding the couple they will appreciate the best culturally diverse cuisine around while they were here.

The sound of their voices flushed Fr. Lighterman out of his room and it wasn't long before he was walking toward their group, crossing the yard in a bee-line for the bishop.

When introductions were over, I saw Sr. Hyacinth pointing in my direction, and noticed the driver shift the suitcases from one arm to the other. It wasn't long before the entire group started heading my way. *Yikes!* Meeting them all at once wasn't something I'd bargained for, so I took the tactical position of slipping out the back door; I knew I would meet the deacons at dinner, Father Lighterman was at every meal, and I was in no hurry to meet the bishop. I left the retreat building while the leaving was good and exited the building by the back door, scurrying down the rear stairs to my hogan.

Safely behind the scenes, it was twenty minutes later when I heard the car engine start again, giving me the impression the bishop was beating a hasty retreat like I had just done.

Deacon Walter was an unassuming person in his thin, short-sleeved plaid shirt. He was much taller than Fr. Lighterman as I compared their heights with a sweeping glance between Fr. Lighterman, who was sitting at the head of the dining table, to Walter sitting next to June near the center. (All meals were shared with them.) Both Walter and June were taller than Father. And with tall Sr. Godwina and short Sr. Evangelista sitting next to each other throwing off my visual curve, I gave up trying to size each one up by the measure of their work boots alone.

A deacon's ministry, I learned over dinner, reaches into many different areas. While deacons are able to distribute communion and conduct prayer services for the sick and dying, they can also witness marriages and may lead reconciliation services. And I was surprised to learn they also proclaim the Gospel and preach among other roles but their main responsibility is to identify with those in need.

"You've come to the right place," I said, "Gallup is filled with needy people."

"So the bishop tells us," Walter said, no doubt picturing the impoverished dwellings off the roadsides. "Especially the rural poor. June and I won't be going out on the reservation much during this trip though, the bishop wants us to devote our time working around the retreat. He has high hopes the retreat will become the spiritual center for the Catholics in Gallup, and be if not profitable, at least it can be sustainable."

"The reservation will come to you," I pointed out, letting them know about Franklin the Navajo and the rocks we were spreading on the paths.

"You hear that, Walter?" June said, her eyes widening in sudden interest. "I told you they aren't all selling artifacts to tourists on the side of the road! We are going to meet our first real Indian and I bet I can get him to tell us about the old ways. And maybe he will explain the meaning behind why the mudstone cliffs are called Baby Rocks[16] we've heard about."

Aware her questions were beginning to stack up like piles of rocks on the side of a hill, I thought, "Poor Franklin, he doesn't know what he's in for."

"Now, June," was all Walter said, curtailing her excited behavior like an experienced lawyer.

"Franklin will keep out of the way," I assured them.

"Oh, but I don't want him to," June argued, anxious to get into his personal store of Indian knowledge like he was a mercantile. "But Walter and I will keep out of the way," June quickly added. "The last thing we want to do is get in the way. We're here to help. If there's anything that needs doing, just let us know and we'll work at it till it's coated over, polished smooth or hammered down," bolstering their reasons for being here. "Like the bishop told us, deacons act like his eyes and ears, so it will be our duty to inform him of any need," showing their intention was to serve, June said nobly, sitting straighter. "Isn't that so, Walter?"

"That's right June…" his sentence finished for him by his wife, letting the rest of his thought to fall to the floor like *Tse Bitai*, rock with wings.[17]

"Our first project, the bishop informed us, will be to paint the hogans. And as the bishop told Sr. Hyacinth, we want to make our time at the retreat center a significant contribution to you and the community," the deacon's wife interrupted.

"You mean staining," I corrected, hoping she wasn't planning on painting over the conflicting textures of natural wood in the timbers and the plaster holding the logs together with a gooey oil-based paint.

"Yes, that's what I meant," she restated. "And if we have time left at the end of summer, the bishop wanted us to start painting the main buildings. I noticed they could use a coat of red paint."

"That's stain too," I said again, figuring she should be made aware of this distinction right from the start in case the bishop, God forbid, had asked them to select the colors for the job.

"You'll find extra stain in the store room under the chapel," Sr. Hyacinth finally informed them to my relief, as I remembered the dried and cracked brushes full of wide splits lying on top of half used cans of stain. If the summer's heat hadn't taken its toll, I was sure disuse had. The rim grooves hardened into hoops of dark alkyd resin prompted a sudden wave of doubt; were Deacon Walter and his wife really as flexible as they put on? Being somewhat older I knew even gates scrape when their hinges rust. I hoped they wouldn't give up after finding out there wasn't enough paint thinner in the whole of Gallup to loosen that dried hardened mess, I thought, while picking at the crusty top of our sugar bowl.

"There is one other thing," June went on, sopping up the last of her gravy with the end of a piece of bread, "we like to say the Office daily and we were wondering if it would be all right if we could use the chapel."

"Certainly," Hyacinth answered, "as long as you schedule your times around the retreat functions, there shouldn't be a problem. Fr. Lighterman says Mass every morning at 8:00, and Srs. Evangelista, Godwina and myself, plus Anne, usually try to meet and recite it together, but it doesn't always work out that way. You're welcome to join us if you want."

When dinner was over Walter and June joined us in a blessing given by Fr. Lighterman for the food we had received. Clinking our coffee cups together in a spirit of bonhomie, we officially welcomed the beginning of their volunteer tour of duty.

Acting as the hewers of wood and drawers of water, the deacon and his wife began the tedious process of scraping and sanding the hogans. The next morning in the bright early light of the New Mexico sun, they rummaged around in the store room under the chapel dragging out their materials. Franklin and I watched as they carted ladders and tools and gallons of stain around us, taking pains not to bestir the rock piles and newly raked pathways. Each day they would break for lunch and fill up on water, which we could see was being recycled on the sweat of their brows.

A work routine emerged. Smoothing the rough wood, patching the hogan joints in the mornings; lunch in the dining room, and back to work again coating the timbers with an almost clear golden tone of stain. Going from hogan to hogan, Walter and June turned out to be very good workers! By 4:00, they would scuttle off tired and sore to their room to clean-up and rest before we would all meet in the chapel to say the Office.

June had always been overly cordial to Franklin (intrigued by him might be a better word) because he was a Navajo, and that kind of obsequious behavior always comes with a red flag; what did she want? Beyond her searching every corner of his knowledge for Indian secrets, Franklin told me confidentially that anyone who was this interested in him and his ancestry was a compliment. He was only too happy to oblige.

It was soon that she revealed her pressing plan. "Why don't we hold our own simulated pow-wow[18] sometime?" she asked, trying not to show how excited she was at the thought. She wasn't aware that in years past a *pow-wow* sometimes referred to a war dance and not always a mysterious get-together, but I was convinced however, she was hoping to see a vision.

"We can build a camp fire and Franklin can tell us about ways of the Navajo. I'm sure Walter will come, he likes to rub off the corners every now and then."

Somedays Bishop Struther would drop by and pick up the husband and wife team and take them on short outings into town. He regularly checked to see how the friends he recommended were doing and if they needed anything; once in a while the three of them went out to dinner.

If I could, I liked to be in the chapel early to settle my mind down and relax before the actual Office began. It was easy to do when no retreatants were there, I would rest my eyes on the timeless beauty of the rise and fall of the hills stretching down to Gallup. I looked forward to these quiet times every afternoon to forgot the hustle and bustle of work.

One day while I was sitting in the chapel, I could hear the sound of muffled talking creep into my awareness. At first I couldn't place where the drone of words was coming from, but shortly the monotony of verbiage grew in intensity and volume and I could tell it was coming from Walter and June's room. It didn't sound like arguing, more like a loud discussion. It was impossible to make out what they were saying if I had wanted to, but Walter's points were definitely louder and longer than June's and it was a sure bet he was finishing his own sentences.

After about a half an hour or so of this, the obtrusive talking would stop and the chapel would again fill with silence. The hall door would quietly open on the right side and the deacon and his wife would enter wearing smiles from ear to ear, as peaceful as you please, ready to recite the hallowed ecclesiastic ceremony known as the Office.

I moved out of the way if they walked close by me and watched them plunk down usually on the front right pew, the pew nearest to their room. I didn't make eye contact with either of them, trying to hide the fact their muffled conversation was somewhat audible in the chapel, as if they could tell this by an ease-dropping look on my face. Being Bishop Struther's personal friends gave them an air of untouchability, as if even suspecting them of indecorous behavior would be a violation of allegiance to the Bishop.

Over the next few days which developed into weeks, daily this loud talking was accompanied by a gradual slow melt down of the recitation of the Office and upcoming rosary; slow, slower, almost to the point of stopping. If Walter announced: *"The Third Glorious Mystery; Descent of the Holy Spirit"* to start the rosary, I would sigh and get ready for another long session. Generally the rosary takes a long time anyway, but it had become a physical and mental strain of drawn out proportions because each decade was accompanied, at his discretion, by a longer and longer meditation on one of the fifteen mysteries. I usually left by about the second decade, and Sr. Hyacinth had long since gone; both of us preferring to finish at our own pace, before dinner.

If Walter sounded like he was slurring his words, friends of the bishop or not, I had the sneaking suspicion talking wasn't the only thing they were doing in their room before the Office. The Deacon was an eloquent speaker, usually, leading us in prayer in a flowery style. But by midsummer, I noticed a change in his speech. Coming from the obviously more relaxed deacon, his articulation had become steadily labored. Listening to him wasn't insightful any more, it had developed into suspenseful anticipation. He wasn't as careful with his enunciations and at times he skidded over expressions, stumbling over words like his tongue was too long and he couldn't keep it from lolling like a dog. Undaunted, he would stop and take great pains to rectify the little slurs in his sentences, repeating the words until they sounded right. He didn't give the appearance of being tipsy because he was cognizant of his lack of crispness; if I didn't think he *may* have been throwing back a few before prayer time, it would have been hard to tell.

June seemed to mellow out too. Her tippled state came with a measure of patience beyond belief, patience that could rival the Virgin Mary. This resignation allowed June to put up with the longest pauses and breaks without becoming antsy, irritated, or even angry. It was as though she had turned a subtle shade of polite pink, never red with fire water. One would never think she was intoxicated, dazed maybe, as if she had just awakened from a long nap aware enough to swat pesky insects off her short-sleeved bloused arms. It was easy to picture her sipping sweet orange liqueur like a southern belle trying to counter the smell of turpentine when cleaning paint brushes. Sitting peacefully in the pew next to her husband, she couldn't have looked more content. Cultured enough to know there is no talking in church, for here and here alone, she quieted her jabbering, a fact which did not go unnoticed by the rest of us and for which we were all thankful.

Summer played out this way. Nursing hangovers or not, Walter and June continued working during the week after the weekend retreat groups had vacated, and one by one the hogans were patched, scraped, sanded and stained. With the addition of the new statue, new rock paths, new finishes on the hogans, and a new staff to boot, by the end of summer St. Francis Retreat really looked spiffy!

As for their tippling, because we weren't *really* sure, no one said anything. Sr. Evangelista didn't bring it up and neither did Sr. Godwina. Fr. Lighterman didn't breathe a reproachful word about it to anyone either and even Sr. Hyacinth courteously looked the other way. I wasn't about to encourage teetotalism on our working guests as a viable alternative. Without conferring, we were of one accord; as long as they were putting stain on the hogans and not each other, it was worth saying the Office at warp speed.

All summer long, it was our little secret.

Chapter 20—Rain Song

When it was dark, in the lowering light of a full moon behind the retreat house, without drums or dancing, we met on the west side of the retreat. Walter, June, Sr. Evangelista, Franklin and myself came together, our shadowy figures slinking silently across the weeded hillside. No retreatants were occupying the large meeting room and it was completely dark. We stopped to look up at the moon reflecting in the separated panels of glass on the conference hall, and watched as a few gray clouds passed from one side of windows over the abrupt interruption of reality of the brick chimney, to connect again in the windows on the other side.

The night was cooling off with hardly a breeze in the air as the heavenly scent of wood smoke floated effortlessly around us. It was a good night for a campfire. June collected a pile of dry twigs and put together a circle of rocks around the pile while I kicked away anything that could catch fire. The five of us sat in a circle and watched as June placed the sticks she'd gathered on top a crumpled piece of newspaper catch fire quickly on the spot, each of us commenting on how much fun it was to camp even if it was in our own back yard. Wanting to make the most of what was left of the summer even in the dark, our faces shone with expectation.

June asked if she could lay a tape recorder to the side of our circle so she could keep our conversation as a remembrance. "I don't see why not," I said looking at Franklin who shrugged his shoulders in indifference. I wondered what we would ever say that would be worth listening to again. Who knew what the night would bring?

Walter began by telling us how he met Bishop Struther. "One of us made it through the seminary, and one of us didn't," he said smiling at June. "We've been friends ever since." June nodded sheepishly as she thought back to their courtship days.

I told them why I wanted to be a volunteer and wanted to learn about Indians, so I chose the retreat in Gallup and did both at the same time.

It was the shank of the evening and now that we had become more closely acquainted, Walter pulled out a large flask from his sweater pocket and offered us a drink. "I *knew* it!" I thought immediately, as he passed the flask around. Thinking the better of it, Franklin declined as did Sister. The situation almost demanded I shouldn't refuse, so I didn't. I screwed off the top, took a swig, passed it to June and let the unknown liquid slide down my throat.

The powerful liquor seemed to pare its way down taking my top layer of tissue with it. "What in God's name *was* that?" I asked, when I got my voice back. I didn't even *want* to know what proof it was.

"Tumbleweed whiskey, the best there is!" the deacon answered with a deep appreciation, holding the flask in front of him using the moon to enlighten the golden alcohol. "If anything will make you see visions, this will," he said, eyeing it affectionately.

In no time at all the five of us were feeling pretty happy, as this authentic rot gut hit our own guts like a petrified rock smashing our inhibitions to smithereens. Catching our enthusiastic behavior, Franklin and Evangelista joined in the revelry too. Once our inner monitors had been loosened and our inner warning systems were ignored, it was amazing how facts, gossip or otherwise, that have been grazing happily for years in the memory will race to the fence once the gate is opened. Stories flowed from us in record time. There never was a lull in the conversation, one of us was always ready with the next story.

By the time the flask was more than three quarters gone, June had found her nerve, and looking directly at Franklin asked, "Franklin, do Navajos still sing rain dances? Do you know any?"

Without answering her with a wordy explanation, I was privileged to hear and see one of the most remarkable occurrences of my life. Franklin began quietly singing in his own language sounding like *heya, hoa, heya hoa,* a rain song. I was aware how special hearing this was in itself, but it didn't hold a candle to what was about to happen. On this seemingly clear night the most improbable thing happened: it started to rain!

Needless to say, we all went wild, congratulating Franklin and shouting our surprise. We were dumbfounded, each of us excitedly reliving the moment when we felt the first drops, reliving how our eyes moved to the fire on hearing the first hissing of the drops on the wood, the telling looks of bewilderment still fixed on our faces, each of us knowing this incredible night was one we would never forget.

Now I don't know anything about meteorology. I can't predict precipitation by the swelling in my joints or tell by the red color of the sky if a delightful day is coming, or forecast a front about to move in by the altitude of swallows (swallows fly low, rain we shall know). All I know is that while I was sitting in dirt on a side of a hill in the dark surrounded by New Mexico's wildlife next to a real native American Navajo Indian, it started to rain!! We were indescribably happy and at one point I called out, "Only in New Mexico!"

The next day, thinking back on our impromptu gathering, I realized what a smart thing it had been for June to bring her tape recorder, because except for the phenomena of the rain, I had a hard time remembering one single story, not to mention the song.

There was little evidence I could use to jolt my memory as I walked through dampened weeds to the location of our campfire: a circle of rocks, the charred remains of our burned out campfire, the lingering smell of smoke in my hair…and one monstrous headache.

Chapter 21—Fanciful Fairies

It was curious to me how I developed such a strong work ethic. Why would I voluntarily do anything that didn't involve play, pleasure or power? I didn't learn this at home, I knew for sure. It had to have been something profound.

Sitting under the big skyhole in the Mother Earth hogan my mother's words came to me predicting, "You'll have more than your share of dishes to do when you're out on your own." How prophetic her words were! If it's true a person is expected to wash about 2.5 million dishes in a lifetime, I estimate my mother washed 10 million, or more. (Still, she had the longest and hardest fingernails I ever saw.) My mother believed childhood was a time for children to spend playing, not working, so consequently I seldom was made to do any housework. She wanted us to remember childhood as a happy-go-lucky existence without the burden of obligations and work.

Then where did my strong work ethic come from? I hadn't been totally useless had I? I did know how to turn on a vacuum and make a bed, and occasionally I set the table. Laundry was different, I did laundry under the watchful eye of a trouble-shooting mother hovering nearby. I ironed, but then again, I was only trusted with hankies and an occasional T-shirt. So I didn't learn the value of work at home. I hadn't been allowed to do the most mundane chore.

I reasoned it must have developed in the monastery. This is where I *really* learned to work because if I didn't finish my work, it was a horrible feeling to have the burden fall on another Sister.

I remembered it was the cook who usually did the cleaning up in the monastery's kitchen, except on a Solemnity such as Christmas when most every plate and pot was dirtied with something from the large meal, then it was permitted for another Sister to offer her help. I could still see them working together in silence hearing nothing but the hasty bangs and clatters.

Washing dishes at the Retreat Center was quite different. It was all hands on deck: separating, stacking, scraping and rinsing, then loading, each job was done by a Sister, and me. Visiting priests, as well as Sisters, would roll up their sleeves and help. Pot detail here was another story. Sr. Hyacinth usually took this disgusting and greasy job on herself like she was preparing for surgery, sticking her gloved hands into the hot soapy water up to her elbows like it was disinfectant, then raising them out of the water again checking for leaks. Confident they were intact, she'd carefully swish apart the floating grime as if she was spreading ribs, disregard her revulsion and slip her hands into the water.

At the retreat work had taken on another dimension for me. After the onslaught of MS even doing the simplest thing became important after losing the use of the right side of my body; leg, arm, hand, and face. Now I was grateful for my every movement. Plugging in a cord really was seeing if my nystagmus (rapid eye movement) had returned and was making the wall socket quiver when I focused on it. Arranging a towel on a rack was a test of my dexterity for my fine motor skills. Walking from room to room was to measure muscle coordination and stiffness. Even the simplest thing like remembering the name of the hogan I walked from and what the next hogan was called, was a cognitive test for my memory. In discussing my day over dinner, I was actually checking to see if I was slurring my words. I made it a point to notice if my smile was smiling up on both left and right sides of my mouth.

After a long day like today I elevated my legs pulling them up on the couch to give them a rest. I knew being here at the retreat, I had something to prove; that I was all the way back to normal and I could trust my body again. Sr. Godwina and Sr. Evangelista went cheerfully about their daily work; my day was a constant assessment of how my body was holding up. It was a subtle but constant reminder.

The last thing I needed to do before leaving today, was check if all the doors were locked. Walking from room to room, I stopped to straighten a rug in a bathroom and was dumbfounded when this harmless motion unleashed an especially meaningful memory.

Not being allowed to do housework had had the reverse effect on me, it made me like to do it, but I had to wait until my mother was out of the house. Then I would clean the bathroom, as best as a five or six year old could. I would wipe out the sink, straighten towels, hang up washcloths, and push clothes that didn't quite make in the gray hamper, inside. When my mother would come home and see the clean bathroom, I'd tell her the same thing every time, "the pixies did it." Knowing how pleased this would make her, was the moment I looked forward to. "The pixies did it," I would say, hardly able to contain my happiness, never letting on I was the one who did the actual cleaning.

I remembered after one such cleaning surprise, a strange thing happened, I had a deep burning in my chest. It wasn't painful, just the opposite. It was an exquisitely good feeling, and it was centered around my heart. I didn't question it because it was such a nice feeling and besides, I thought everyone felt it. If God feels like this, it will be wonderful passing into heaven.

No wonder I was drawn to St. John of the Cross and his references to fire: enkindled with love, fire of love, Divine fire of love, *Kindled in love with yearnings* (*Ascent of Mount Carmel*, Book I, chapter XIV), and his entire last work, *Living Flame of Love*. Just *thinking* about how I surprised my mother, would bring back the same sensation.

Eventually though, over time the feeling began to weaken, and at some point it went away altogether, leaving an indelible mark in my memory.

I wished I could feel it here and now in the hogan but pleasing Sr. Hyacinth didn't have the same emotional oomph as pleasing my mother did.

I wanted to check anyway…I walked into one of the bathrooms and stood there a second. It had recently been cleaned but noticing a smudge on the mirror, I tore off a few sheets of tissue from the roll and began to wipe at the smear. Suddenly I saw myself as a little girl cleaning happily, eager for her mother to come home so she could again give credit the pixies.

Hoping to feel the burning again, I stopped abruptly to see if the virtuous feeling had returned. Nothing, besides feeling a little headachy from inhaling odors left by cleaning products. Saddened, I realized the years must have tarnished my soul like the mirror because I have never felt it since. A light went on in my mind. Was discrediting my actions and ascribing them to pixies an act of self-denial? Is that what produced the burning? Had this been the origin and basis of my strong work ethic all along? If so, I hadn't been far off the mark in my thinking, the pixies really *did* do it!

Chapter 22—Breaking Through

"Franklin's had an accident," I heard Sr. Hyacinth yell out the window as she slowed the car toward me in the retreat yard. "He's in the hospital. Climb in, Anne, we're on our way to see him."

Sliding into the back seat next to Sr. Evangelista, I asked, "What happened?"

"We don't know, his brother was tight-lipped about the whole thing. All he would say was Franklin had an accident and was in an Indian hospital, but I don't think his brother knows as much English as Franklin so maybe he couldn't tell me more if he wanted to," Hyacinth remarked with a resigned look. "Like I always say, you have to expect the unexpected here in Indian country."

Tall Sr. Godwina bent her head a little so I could hear her but her voice was lost in the lurching and jostling of the car on the uneven surface of the retreat exit. Unable to make out a word she said, I smiled at her anyway like I'd heard every word.

I was actually thinking about Franklin. Boy, was I ever glad we hadn't coerced him into taking a drink with us at our get-together! I felt guilty anyway, remembering how my father with his own alcohol problem would watch a football or baseball game *perfectly sober*, but was no match against the onslaught of non-stop beer commercials like brainwashing. By half-time or the seventh inning stretch he was out the door heading for a liquor store. I hoped just the smell of alcohol didn't have the same effect on Franklin and set him off. I would feel terrible if thought if I had inadvertently caused him to think, "Oh, I *looove* that Tumbleweed Whisky too," toying with the thought until he couldn't resist seeing if it really *was* as good as he remembered.

We joined the main highway and made a right turn taking us north into Gallup and even though the car noise was diminished by the smoother road, we were a silent group wondering what could have happened to Franklin. 'We were almost finished scattering the rock on the paths,' I thought, hoping I hadn't pushed him too hard causing a heart attack or some other hidden heart condition to surface. I hadn't asked him to do anything I wouldn't do myself, I knew, reassuring myself again.

Even with Hyacinth's fast pace it still seemed we were taking forever to get into town. With little to focus on on either side of the road but collections of dried weeds, I thought it would have been nice to walk in holding a bouquet of flowers to cheer him.

Finally, from the fast motion of the highway we moved onto residential streets and wove our way through a blur of old one-story homes. Regular homes with front lawns, garages and children's bikes on the lawns.

At last we were here, our car slowed and stopped at the visitor section of the hospital's parking lot. "I want to tell the three of you," Sr. Hyacinth warned, as she turned to face the back seat, "an Indian hospital is different than the hospitals you're used to. Gallup is a ethnic and cultural mix, with the Native American culture most prominent, of course, you'll see differences I assure you. But on the whole, the care is quite good. If the girls need a comprehensive assessment before they are placed with us, we bring them here. Or if they need nutritional counseling, or even a couple of times to get walk-in emergency care, they come here. It's comforting to know help is so close, especially since I'm stationed at the retreat house and Celeste is on her own.

While some Navajos choose hospitals, the girls tell me when disorder is in a Navajo's life, sometimes a traditional medicineman[19] is sought using herbs and prayers as a cure.

The closer we came to actually entering the hospital, the more nervous I became. Not about going into this hospital, it was any hospital. My own hospital stay hadn't been that long ago with my first acute episode of MS. It was a time I didn't want to be reminded of and here I was about to enter the antiseptic white-sheeted world of sickly people again, walking straight into their miasmic influences. I already had one disease, I didn't want to catch another.

We pulled into the hospital's parking lot. I took one last long breath of clean outside air, determined not to breathe very much during the remainder of the visit. With the three Sisters, we went through the heavy plate glass doors of the entrance.

Glancing around the lobby though, I saw it was just like any other hospital, clean and orderly with tiled walls, and I let myself inhale deeply. Sr. Hyacinth asked about Franklin's room number from the admitting clerk, #347, and the four of us moved toward the elevator. We stood like freight going from floor to floor. Listening to the sqeaking and straining of the elevator's guide rails as they hoisted us upwards, I inwardly wondered if they had enough pull to make it past the next half floor with all of us. I certainly didn't want to be confined in this small compartment filled with other people's lingering germs just looking for a host to latch onto any longer than I had to. As a reminder not to touch anything, I stuck my hands in my pockets.

Thoughts came winging back to me of my own hospital stay. I remembered the emergency room doctor told me he had treated a patient right before me who had broken all of his knuckles when he held onto the roll bar of a jeep as it rolled it several times; my hands involuntarily tightened into fists.

Crammed into this elevator I recalled something else the ER doctor had told me, that he had completed his residency here, at this very hospital! Suddenly I felt a kinship which awakened a confidence in this place and its treatments. I felt at peace knowing Franklin was in good hands and I stopped wondering when the elevator had its last safety inspection. Hearing the three dings announcing our floor, we waited for the door to automatically open, timely and smooth, like I now trusted it would.

We pushed from the elevator and found ourselves in a long unventilated hallway filled with the smell of disinfectant. A small number of patients lay on gurneys in various stages of health along the wall. Visitors were unfortunately conducting their visits here out in the open with patients who didn't have a room. This was inconvenient to say the least for them, because I knew what an imposition it was to feel bad in public and having to wear a cheerful face for passerbys.

While we walked, I thought of several other reasons for the gurneys to be here; maybe the patients were waiting for orderlies; or they could have been waiting for a room to be cleaned; patients here were being taken into surgery in another ward; maybe they were waiting to be dismissed; or the hospital was just to small.

We wound our way around patients and guests which paused their flow of Navajo conversation the closer we came to each group. It was surprising how many people knew Sr. Hyacinth as she extended her hand in healing touches of support to those that offered, inviting stares and inquisitive looks plus a few "Hi, Sisters" as we passed. Finally we came to room #347 and walked through the open door to find Franklin lying on his back with his left foot in a cast.

"What happened Franklin?" Hyacinth asked even before we were all in the room. "Are you all right?"

"Yah te hey, Sister," Franklin spoke softly, obviously under the influence of pain pills but not forgetting his manners. "Don't worry Sister. It's nothing. I feel fine," looking mildly surprised at her concern. Then noticing the rest of us standing at the foot of his bed, he smiled at the novices and apologized to me, "Sorry I can't help any more spreading the rocks, I broke my ankle."

"Don't worry about the rocks," relieved it was only a broken bone instead of something more serious. "How did you break it?"

He looked at his ankle. "Well ah, it's a funny thing. I was stepping out of my brother's truck, and he thought I was all the way out, and I was out…but only part of me, all but my left leg. The truck kept going with me in it, half in and half out. Then I heard a loud crack and…"

"That's okay Franklin, we get the picture," I cut in, beginning to feel squeamish. It didn't take much to make me queasy and hearing about anything like solid bone mass snapping was enough to make me have an overall feeling of weakness in my entire body.

Sr. Hyacinth broke the dismal mood in the room by asking, "Franklin, had you been drinking?"

He didn't seem the least annoyed, apparently expecting the question. I had the impression his reply would be, would be, "Of course I was drinking. Do you think I am this clumsy when I'm sober?"

Politely responding to her, he said instead, "Sister, I can not tell you a lie. Yes, I was drinking."

"Now Franklin, you see what drinking brings to you? Accidents and misfortune. What do you have to say for yourself?"

"Nothing Sister," his eyes moving to his foot again to avoid eye contact with her. "Only I promise I won't drink any more."

"…or any less," I finished, thinking of one of my father's favorite lines. We never found the humor in it then, and by the look on Hyacinth's face, she didn't now.

"Indians seem to have a harder time controlling their liquor, isn't that right Franklin?" she asked, the smile gone from her face.

Not knowing if this was true or not I knew she was trying to make the point that he shouldn't drink at all. The evils of drinking was an indomitable uphill battle. Good luck trying to get *that* in his head, Sr. Hyacinth, I thought.

With a sheepish grin, not wanting to pursue what he thought was a pointless conversation, he turned his face away from Hyacinth and toward the novices and me and changed the subject by asking in a low voice if any of us had ever broken a bone.

"I broke a finger once when a horse threw me," Sr. Evangelista led off, holding out a crooked little finger as proof.

"I severely bruised my right forearm once but because the ulna wasn't broken, I didn't get to have a cast, only a brace," Sr. Godwina added, sounding disappointed.

I told her I thought having an arm imprisoned in a cast would be an accurate keepsake for those four years, a fitting souvenir describing high school.

"Plus a cast can act like a plaster yearbook with everyone signing it," she enthused.

"You know what St. John of the Cross says about breaking a bone, don't you?" I asked, "God is increasing the person's spirit."

"Did it ever happen to you?" Franklin asked, in a misery loves company attitude.

"No, I never had a broken bone, I said, "but I'll never forget a strange thing that happened to me one afternoon. I had passed this lake many times before, but why my sister and I decided this particular afternoon to stop, drive in and see it, I don't know."

"It was a weekday and only a few families were there camping or picnicking even though it was a bright sunny day. The lake was surrounded by grassy hills but before we began looking around, we wanted to locate a rest room. Driving toward the camping area we found the outside facilities on the side of the road, outhouses. I was wearing an expensive pair of sunglasses I didn't want to break or lose so when I opened the wooden door, I stood on the stoop with the daylight flooding in, and looked for a safe place to lay them. There was a ledge on the left side and before I shut the door I placed the glasses very carefully on the ledge. No sooner had I done this, I heard a woman screaming for help.

We followed the calls and found the excited woman caring for her daughter in the playground who had broken her arm by flinging off a swing and we took the pair to the ranger station at the entrance for help.

"This is the part I can't understand, when I went back to get my sunglasses, I opened the door and saw one of the arms was broken too, like it had been snapped in half! How could that have happened, especially after taking such care setting them down?" wondering out loud.

"You probably weren't as careful as you thought, that's all," Sr. Hyacinth said, taking the eerieness out of it with common sense.

"Yes, that's probably it," the novices agreed, finding comfort in the familiar explanation.

"No," Franklin said. "Your strong feelings broke your glasses. What you were feeling on the inside, came out on the outside. Your feelings were strong. Too strong for your body to take on. They came out in the glasses."

We stood there staring bemusedly at Franklin trying to make sense of what he said.

He continued, "Like watching someone fall and break their wrist, you might do the same to relieve your bad feelings about it. Or like when you pray for good health for me, you are also praying for yourselves. Feelings act in these ways when they are strong."

Breaking the mood, Hyacinth said, "If that's the case, I hope you get well and stay well!" and we all laughed.

Squeezing his good hand good-bye, Sr. Hyacinth muttered a final Yah te hey and we all shuffled out the door.

Sr. Evangelista led the way back into the busy hall interrupting conversations of well-wishers again, family members curiously turning to look at the Sisters in their habits. I was grateful my attire looked somewhat like what they were wearing, blending in with my almost-clean jeans and not-so-clean tennis shoes.

Once outside, I took long cleansing breaths before closing the car door behind me. We moved through the residential tracts and onto the highway with the beauty of the distant hills surrounding us again. I had plenty to occupy my mind during the ride home: the look of the Indians in the hallway caring for their loved ones, Franklin's broken ankle and the awkward way he fell while drunk, Sr. Evangelista falling off a horse herself, and especially Franklin's unusual degree of prayer, to make the ride home go by quickly.

I didn't expect to find murmuring fountains in the lobby in this hospital. I didn't even expect to find spacious wards. And I really didn't expect to come away with an overall positive picture of the facility. But like Hyacinth says, 'you have to expect the unexpected here in Indian country', even if it is turns out to be a fascinating surprise.

Chapter 23—In Hot Pursuit

Had the Navajo Nation been rubbing off on my intuition the moment I stepped off the train? The locality itself contains forces of power, strength, urgency and energy so why wouldn't I be caught up in its ministrations? Learning about its Great Seal depicting a yellow sun shining from the east on four sacred mountains: Mt. Blanca, Mt. Taylor, Mt. Hesperus and San Francisco Peak, with the four directions represented as colors; east as White Shell, west as Yellow Abalone, north as jet Black, and south as Turquoise, I couldn't help feel as a newcomer, the natural beauty was infiltrating my being with the sole purpose of drawing me closer.

The more I admired the calm endurance and steadiness of the landscape, the more I found myself filled with the subtle effects of peace and calmness and patience.

I began noticing how scents of the Southwest filling the gorges with the perfume of desert flowers stilled my disquieting thoughts more effectively than a fragrant soothing balm.

I watched cloud shadows cross over fields and patches of shade move above the heat soaked soil allowing insight to break through in streams of brilliant rays of light.

I saw clumps of dirt blasted by wind shift evenly into red plains, and hills dotted with thick-limbed brittlebush cactus thrust their limbs skyward in ever-changing transformation.

I recalled tufts of branches swaying in trees together with boulders balanced precariously on bluffs holding steadfast against the horizon.

I was aware of ultra violet rays beaming over all this scenic beauty created afterglows of warm light entered my awareness as breathtaking views.

Does natural beauty awaken my attention through rainbows, wild fauna, and sacred mountains? Does beauty stimulate the spirit and heighten spirituality? Was this what was bringing back my extraordinary experiences in the incredible fish tale, the unwelcome camping intruder, the burning feeling the pixies caused?

Were New Mexico's mystical bonds of beauty opening new dimensions in my consciousness? I didn't know for sure, but I was hot on the trail.

Chapter 24—Waste Not, Want Not

There was a good chance I was becoming spoiled and there was nothing I could do about it, it came with the territory. Positioned behind three square meals a day, in between serving generous portions of tasty meals to retreatants, I had the dubious honor of accepting the fact that my gravy boat, had indeed, come in.

As a person trying to live as a Trappistine in theory, the retreat lifestyle did present something of a problem. Though I didn't receive a weekly pay check, it was a life where good measure may not have been running over, it had least been pressed down and shaken together; just about the antithesis of the half-starved underfed monks I'd heard about during the refectory readings at the monastery I wanted to emulate; having more than I needed was not my ideal way to live. But before I could live up to the faultless perfection of monastic practices I had in my mind's eye, I recalled a telling incident that brought my highfalutin ideals down a notch.

It happened one afternoon when I was still in the monastery which humbled me like a slap in the face. It involved the entire ascetic group of nuns and taught me I was in no position to judge.

Tapping her teaspoon against a water glass, Reverend Mother Eleanor, the monastery's superior, announced a couple of the abbey's benefactors had asked if they could prepare a special side dish for us. Due to their donations in the past, and not wanting to do anything to jeopardize future contributions (I was sure), the husband and wife cooking team were allowed to prepare a gourmet dish for all of us in the guest house where they were staying. Smiling broadly, Rev. Mother smacked her fingers against her lips giving us a sign of 'bon appetite'.

When 12:00 dinner time neared, we were seated around the refectory table anxious to experience the mouth-watering dish. We watched as the side door opened and the two visiting cooks entered carrying a large pot filled with some sort of gastronomical delight and placed it on the stove. They fiddled (in silence) over the pot with salt shakers stirring in last minute seasonings like proud grandparents grinning from ear to ear. When it at last met their approval, they took their seats at the guest table and waited to watch our expressions as we sampled their toothsome delight.

After Rev. Mother said grace, out of politeness she motioned them to serve themselves first. I watched with anticipation as they dipped a large ladle into the pot filling their soup bowls in one try. They were beaming when they took their seats across the room, close to our chaplain Mac, as they readied to monitor our expressions closely as we ate. They genuinely wanted to share their favorite dish with Sisters who'd think they'd died and gone to heaven when they tasted their flavorful food.

As the newest novice, it was my turn next to serve myself behind our guests. Walking all the way around the long refectory table I tried to distinguish a savory aroma that would give me an indication of what the pot contained, but I wasn't able to detect a thing. Hungrily I closed in on the pot. Picking up a pot holder, I lifted the lid and to my amazement (and revulsion), I saw a bubbling pot was full of onions! Big ones and little ones, some the size of pearls and some as big as golf balls stewing in their own juice. *Onion soup!* How could they think food fit for the Middle Ages was also fit for us too? Assuming it was a delicacy somewhere in the world, I thought, here goes nothing, and plunged the ladle into the mix, trying my best to keep a 'it looks delicious' look on my face for their benefit. I lifted the ladle full of little round onions in various shapes, pea size, marble size, ping-pong ball size; concentric edible bulbs floating amid fleshy transparent coverings. The rest of the community served themselves after me.

I have always been a lover of onions, the stronger the better; onions in tuna with mayonnaise, onions alone on a wedge of cheese, onions diced into just about everything, so as I was carrying my bowl back to my place I looked forward to my first mouthful and thought I'd really enjoy this unusual fare. The first spoonful was good and I smiled widely, and looking across the room, I gave the cooks a thumbs up in appreciation.

The first spoonful *was* good. It was after about the fifth I started having trouble and it wasn't long before I realized I had already reached my onion limit. At some point into an onion meal, the very thought of the large amount still to be eaten is enough to turn the stomach. I looked at the other novices, who I noticed were taking their time bringing their spoons to their mouths as well, in fact, we all were. Not wanting to be wasteful, we tried to eat as much as we could, but after a quick and inconspicuous hand sign from the Novice Mistress of 'stay' which had a variety of meanings: remain, wait, endure, rest, to name a few; in this case it meant '*leave* what you can't possibly eat'.

I suppose it was the right thing to do, but in the back of my mind were nagging doubts, should I have forced myself to eat the remaining onions in my bowl? What would have been the spiritual way to act? Then again, making myself sick wasn't spiritual either. This was what I was pondering as I sat staring into the lumps of bad tasting globosity remaining in my soup bowl. I waited for the visiting cooks to leave so as not to insult them when I made my way to the table in the back of the room to fill up on peanut butter and bread. This confirmed it then, I was in no position to judge spiritual behaviors.

But Gallup had an unusual way of leading me all the way around and out the other end of a full circle to remind me of my shortcomings.

"Santa's on his way, and we're going to head him off at Sandia Pass!" Sr. Hyacinth called as she opened the car door and climbed behind the wheel. It was the excited tone in her voice that raised my attention. I was always ready for a little diversion away from the practical operations of the Retreat Center.

It was December so Hyacinth's statement about Santa did make some sense, and was typical of Hyacinth who always seemed to have surprises up her sleeve, but that's what made Hyacinth, Hyacinth. She had a strong will that wouldn't back down but could back *you* down; her red-colored cheeks had something to do with this, giving the impression she was holding her temper and could blow at any moment, it was better not to chance it. For the most part, as I observed her in her dealings with people over the months, she was usually right.

Knowing it was always adventurous to go with Sister *wherever* she went, I shook my head up and down like an excited dog, happy to be going along for the ride. Walking to the community's car, I also knew once the cool clear air was streaming over our vehicle carrying scents of the southwest with it, I would have a hard time resisting the urge to stick my head out the window like a four legged friend too. Instead, I resigned myself to draping my head over the front seat so I'd be able to hear conversation.

Never having been to Albuquerque before, I welcomed the opportunity to see museums I'd heard about, some housing 20,000 BC artifacts, and others more well known like the atomic bomb museum. Maybe take in a memorial, look at authentic Native American costumes, walk through historic places this town was sure to have.

Straightening her veil in the mirror Hyacinth added, "We're targeting those most in need this Christmas." This too, was not a surprising statement coming from a missionary Sister, optimistically confident the community's indigent could be straightened out as easily as she straightened her veil.

Sr. Godwina, summoned by Hyacinth's call, closed the office door and walked over to our waiting car, her sandals slapping their way across the rocks on the paths. She mirrored Hyacinth in black veil and habit. I always avoided sitting in the front seat in case they wanted to discuss private community plans, finances, or road directions because of their *Sister* status. Pushing a car pillow out of the way, I climbed in the back seat and prepared myself for the three hour plus car ride to Albuquerque. As soon as Godwina was settled in the passenger seat, I felt the car lurch and we moved down the decline on the driveway and we were on our way.

It didn't take long before we were at the outskirts of Gallup. On the open road with the desert roaming endlessly flat and low on both sides of the highway, I settled back to enjoy the scenery. I could hear the Sisters conversing in an informal chat, but it wasn't until Sr. Hyacinth momentarily turned her head so her voice would carry back to me that I heard, "You hear that Anne?"

"No, I didn't," I yelled back, pulling myself up closer to the front.

"I spoke with a Sr. Elaine last night," Hyacinth shouted. "She's not one of our Order. She's with another one. They provide domestic…" her words were lost in the noise of a passing truck. "She told me now would be a good time to come and collect."

"What?" I screamed.

Sr. Godwina took over. Scooting herself around to face me she said, "Ever hear of a food bank?"

"No, what's that?"

"People who aren't in need usually never hear about them. The convent where I was stationed before had one nearby. It's unfortunate, but people object to having them in their neighborhoods."

"Why?"

Speaking loudly and in short bursts, Godwina quickly filled me in. "They attract the wrong element, down and out types; homeless, disabled, sick. They provide food to the hungry. In some respect food banks are underground operations. People don't like to advertise the fact that they don't have money for food. They avoid being seen. They don't look directly at people. Heaven forbid they should see someone they know."

"I'll remember that," I said, making a mental note not to stare. "But if people are going hungry, why aren't there more of them?"

Halfway turning her head to face me, Sr. Hyacinth trying to talk over the wind whistling from the window, said, "Oh you'd be surprised. They're out there, you just don't know where."[20] And taking a big gulp of air, she continued, "It's Sr. Elaine's job to distribute what people donate. You know, bread, flour, rice, staples. You'll see."

"You mean it's all donated?"

"Most of it. The government supplies some, like peanut butter, and cheese occasionally," ending her explanation. I went back to looking at the wide range of open land as it passed. We all did.

The first thing I noticed about Albuquerque was how flat it was, almost as flat as Tucson, if it wasn't for scenic Sandia peak pressing its way into view. With an elevation of more than 10,000 feet, I was told there was an aerial tramway used during summer and fall that gives an amazing view of about half of New Mexico from the top.

"Don't forget the Sangre de Cristo mountain range to the east of the city," Hyacinth added, pointing her hand in an easterly slant. "It's known for its beautiful red color," prompting me to look harder out the car window. "And the Rio Grande on the west side of the city is well-known for its slow meandering beauty, and although most of it is underground, it waters the whole central valley. In spring and summer, on each side of the road, you can see a beautiful fertile sight of fields and orchards."

Quite a difference from the plain hard desert floor I saw now to picturing it in a lush verdant green cover. No wonder the Indians, the Spaniards and the Mexicans were always fighting over it.

"Still settlers were able to run irrigation ditches and sow fields," clarified Hyacinth, adding that the Villa of Albuquerque was named after the viceroy, Fernandez de la Cuerva, Duke of Albuquerque in 1704. "But it was Catholic missionaries that first settled in the area in the 1600s," stating these facts about the early missionaries, not only in a knowledgeable tone, but in a familial one as well.

The second thing that caught my eye as we drove slowly over the clean streets were the numerous bunches of red strands of chili peppers hanging to dry on doorways and windows, over alley gates and under eaves. The chilies hadn't been attached in a haphazard manor, they had been arranged with great precision and care. The end result were works of art consisting of sometimes 500 firmly fastened fruits on a strand. They were formed in irregular shapes—teardrop shapes and pear, cylindrical, or circular, hanging in different lengths in bunches neatly secured in foot long lengths to two yards pulled together. Chilies the size of cherry tomatoes on top, followed by fatter radish size, with the longer cigar sizes hanging at the bottom in creative displays.

Hyacinth explained that these chilies were called *ristras* and were what gave the spice to New Mexico's food. I told her I knew this for a fact after accepting a taste of one of these chilies from one of their girls soon after I arrived, adding, "Never again!"

Albuquerque was not the adobe lined streets I was expecting but I did see a slower pace metropolis with boys walking across the street wearing cowboy boots, older Indian women wearing bright colors sitting peacefully against newish buildings. And rooftops that were lined with *luminarias*[21] that I was told were lunch-sized brown paper bags strategically placed about a residence or business a few yards apart, each bag filled with enough sand to stabilize a votive candle. At night during the Christmas season the candles were lit giving a decorative and festive atmosphere. "You'll see tonight," Hyacinth said.

"That is what happens to people when they decide to cross the desert mid-day in the summer," Sister warned, pointing to the two cattle skulls hanging on the front of a Rattlesnake Museum & Gift Shop.

"We'll remember that," Godwina and I said wryly, appreciating her attempt at dry humor.

It was well after lunch so before we went on to the Food Bank, we decided to stop for lunch. By-passing the fast food places, we chose a modest restaurant serving authentic southwestern food which, I was sure, must have been prepared with *ristras*. As long as they were cut up, diced or mashed in, they added a gusto, a southwestern twang to the food, and not the fire I remembered. The food was delicious.

The Food Bank wasn't a warehouse at all; it didn't even have a sign out in front. It was located inside a regular family home that looked like it had been built in the fifties. It had a side entrance hidden by two large overgrown bushes on both sides that obscured visitors from the view of the rest of the neighborhood. An arch opened on a low entryway where visitors waited surrounded by yellowed flowered wall-paper above worn dingy linoleum giving the impression it was a high trafficked area.

As we followed Sr. Hyacinth into the house I saw rooms filled with food, some rooms literally piled to the roof with stuffed burlap sacks and boxes. It was a sprawling ranch style house with many small rooms and the food had been separated accordingly; canned goods, flour, oatmeal, peanut butter, sugar etc.

In one of these rooms I happened to see an Anglo woman off by herself choosing items in an unhurried manner. I only had a glimpse of her as I was following tall Srs. Hyacinth and Godwina and they were moving at a fast clip. The woman had shoulder length brown straggly hair, snarled on the side I saw.

Sr. Elaine greeted us with the subject at hand by letting us know what was available for us to take and what had been marked in advance for certain groups. And moving to one side and pushing doors ajar so we could see the cardboard "do not take" signs holding items, she commented how the local market dropped off a large amount of groceries in time for Christmas and told us the foodbank received nearly double the amount of donations in December, so we could take what we needed, telling us the spirit of human kindness is very strong during the holidays.

Sr. Elaine had a seraphic smile, a preferred quality for someone to have who deals with the down and possibly out. There was a calmness about her which exuded an attitude of *there's enough for everyone*, giving the assurance there was. Aware people were waiting for what could be the first meal they had that day, her kind smile helped to mitigate a patron's dire circumstances. I imagined her in her former life as being a caregiver, possibly a nurse asking patients to "step right this way and roll up their sleeve," while handing out tissues for children to wipe any tears.

Sr. Elaine continued to explain that while some Sisters regularly pick up food to distribute weekly, other Sisters came only when there was an urgent need. "Much of the food that is dropped off is surplus, so there is no telling what the day will bring, canned goods, jars of mayonnaise, even stuffed animals. It's kind of exciting to see; God knows what's needed and it's uncanny to see the very thing that is needed dropped off the same week."

"It would be," I agreed, but wondering what they did when nothing was donated that week. (I was having a hard time imagining hunger with our lunch lying heavy in my stomach.)

I asked about the woman I saw. "She was in one of the rooms; what would she do if nothing was dropped off that week?"

"Oh that's Maggie. She's been coming around here regular like. She's fallen on hard times but she'll get back on her feet again. She has that kind of spirit. Foodbanks are made for people like her. It's true what they say, most people are one check away from being homeless, and that's true in Maggie's case."

Hearing the faint sound of paper rippling as Maggie carried her bags toward us in the hall, Sr. Elaine switched the topic telling us about the foodbank's charitable distribution of food. "We won't let anybody go away hungry," she said. "We can always find something, even if it's from our own larder."

We pretended we were busy for Maggie's benefit, acting as if we hadn't been talking about her. Sr. Godwina and I opened a few shopping bags and busily began to fill them with a variety of cans.

Maggie walked into the room with her loaded shopping bags. Without staring, we glanced her way. She wasn't much older than me, I thought, and close up I saw her hair was knotted. There were light smudges of dirt on her face and arms. Turning toward her, her clothes looked wrinkled and had the drab look of needing a wash. It was understandable when I thought about it, why should she put quarters into slots to fill a washing machine, when she could lay quarters on a counter to buy a loaf of bread? Anyone would choose the same.

She flashed us a placid smile as she readjusted her grip on the bags and said, "Thank you Sister" to Elaine and left carrying her food.

We muttered polite good-byes after her, but her fleeing figure was already gone. She brought new meaning to John Bradford's quote, "There, but for the grace of God, go I."

On my first trip to Albuquerque I saw first-hand how a foodbank touched the life of a needy woman who was down on her luck and needed food and how she was able to leave with enough provisions to get her at least through the month. I learned that some restaurants and supermarkets, instead of discarding food for whatever reason, cooperated with foodbanks by passing along this food.

I came away with the strong sentiment how morally special the people were who made it a point to give of themselves and remember those who didn't have enough to eat. In my heart I knew there must be a special place in heaven for generous people like these who understood they would be blessed in considering the poor.

On the drive home, the lone figure of Maggie moving from room to room gathering food, half hidden by the stacks of food was disturbing. Was it because she was so close to my own age I found her unsettling? Or was I bothered by the fact I knew she had to go without food at times? Turning these questions over in my mind, I suddenly thought, *no*.

Up ahead in the spreading darkness my eyes picked up an unusual sight. I could see hundreds of luminarias lighting the dark streets of Albuquerque outlining walkways, edging curbs, bordering rooftops in an up-and-down procession of illumination. And as I watched these twinkling lights of the city sparkle brighter and brighter, it was as if my intuition had brightened too. I finally realized what was eating away at me and it had little to do with another person's underprivileged situation and everything to do with my own because somehow I knew, that whether they had been pickled, soggy or crunchy, Maggie would have eaten all the onions.

Chapter 25—Emperor of the Dump

To some people dumping garbage isn't a high point in their life, but it was in mine; I loved to go to the dump! One of my favorite activities at the retreat was when Sr. Hyacinth brought the white pickup truck so we could make an expedition to the local dump. Living so far out of town we didn't have a regular trash pickup so we had to wait for different unscheduled intervals when the city combined our pick up with that of the nearby parishes', but when our own ongoing yard work and cleaning had grown into an unusually large unsightly mound on the side of road, then Hyacinth would decide it was time to bring the truck around so we could haul it away ourselves.

It didn't look like a regular dump with an attendant tallying up each load we dropped off. It was more of a place where the local people had decided they would bring their refuse and everyone somehow knew where it was. It wasn't out-of-control dumping but reasonable piles of everyday-living dumping because people here burned most of what they didn't need for heat, which kept their throw away items to a minimum.

There were no signs of course, Hyacinth had been there many times before and knew the general direction to drive. I knew we were getting closer when I began seeing various stages of decomposition on the sides of the road; flat tires, springs that had lost their coil, pieces of indestructible plastic, candle ends, and smoking pipes that had lost their pull. One carrion-eating bird was picking at a little offal it had found.

Launching garbage off the back of the truck was fun, no doubt, as I pulled myself up on the opened ledge of the pickup. Hoisting myself in with the leaves, clippings and other odd scouring from the retreat, I stepped in between the branches and loose piles of mildewy white leaves and picked up a rake we'd burrowed in the heap. Flinging off the top layer of the messy jumble, I dragged and scraped the bed of the truck as I flung.

Sr. Hyacinth struggled out of the truck and tightened an apron around her like it was a mantle of honor, pulling the crucifix hanging around her neck safely out of the way and began tossing anything she could reach off the pick-up. Even though she was in black habit and veil, if there was the need throw trash, then she threw trash.

What really made this dump special was a rock formation that was grotesque and beautiful at the same time. Technically, it could be classified as a monolith because it *was* a single large stone. It only split into four chunks on top, but it was still all connected with four separate very dark brown-reddish heads attached to a base of practically white sedimentary quartz. It was impossible to account for the colors in this rock. The contrast was remarkable.

The rock was an enigma for me. How could wind, rain and snow whiten the base while deepening the redness in the stony hairstyles at the top on the same time? It must have taken years to sculpt such a bizarre formation. Rugged and chiseled, it was beautiful in its uniqueness but also grotesque in its strangeness because the dark heads looked like they had grown out of the thick bone at the base of pale sandstone. I pulled my eyes across the four thick stone hair pieces and over the wrinkles in their foreheads, down the accordion-like thickness of their necks; I stood back and admired it every dumping day.

All this picturesque beauty in the middle of nowhere was going to waste. I knew its days were numbered. Like four jewels set on a stone, I knew the emperor of the dump would eventually meet an ignominious end by crumbling away until only the base remained as it passed beyond the world of existence like a pilgrim. Its delicate balance would run down its necks to its base like it had been desecrated by vandals. New Mexico's relentless heat and icy downpours would act as its karma in a visible cause and effect in the insensible passing from sand to another representation. Helpless, the heads accepted their fate, as they had earlier incarnations connected and bound for eternity together like some mythological creature.

The first and biggest head was turned and faced in a completely different direction from the other heads giving the impression it was trying to change its destiny. Its primordial sense of smell was exaggerated by its unusually large brown and red nose that was out of proportion to its face, like it had grown in its search for a higher consciousness. And the slight color gradation on each of the heads reminded me of the stages of its transition.

Going to the dump for me was a meditation. Where most people would approach with caution fish entrails, broken lamps, and bottomless buckets, the emperor of the dump beckoned me. The more I visited, the more I began to see New Mexico as the *Land of Enchantment* was actually an enchantress using its shapes to charm and coerce the onlooker to enter into the spirit of its unique rock formations.

At times my imagination would involuntarily fashion indistinct dream-like configurations brought on by the energy emanating from the rocks, much like I was looking at blotted patterns of spilled ink. But the inkblots here are not on printed cards but on the jutting and jagged ledges and towering cynosures of balancing rocks. The forms of smooth rock suggest interpretations that split open archetypes like broad arrows allowing a new way of thinking to emerge.

New Mexico's heart of rock reshapes perceptions by stretching the mind in wonder, tantalizing the imagination and encouraging the creative faculty naturally without effort, passing abstractions easily through the mind by bewitching the unaware observer under the orange red sun in the sky.

Chapter 26—Field of Vision

Our horseback riding escapade started when a retreatant discovered Sr. Evangelista was as much a lover of horses as she. Now there are horse people, and then there people who live and breathe horses almost like it had been bred into them and when two people like this meet it is better to back out of the way because any riding experience you may have had will be pale in comparison to their knowledge and love of horses. It didn't take long to realize these were two such people.

At her invitation we met at Jane's Lazy Pine ranch. We turned right on the highway traveling south and went under a decorative metal arch with an outline of a pine tree leaning on its side welded on top, and followed a long straight dirt road lined with ground-in parts of weeds that once were tiny yellow flowers; out of harm's way, their intact counterparts could be seen growing on the surrounding fields among shoots of cactus.

Behind this, and spreading down from the side of the hill was a solid wall of dovetailing pine trees. This mixture of cactus and pine at the elevation of 7,000 feet, not extremely high but not a low basin either, looked as if both species couldn't decide where it should be growing, so each genus braced itself for whatever the weather blew its way and began growing where it was in a thorough confusion, not knowing whether to remain dormant or spring into life.

Sr. Evangelista drove us in to the ranch stopping at a corral that was lined with cowboys straddling old splintered wooden posts. They were an interesting lot in their jeans and leg chaps; mostly Anglo, a few Navajo, but all were real cowboys.

Jane galloped to us as we pulled up to watch the action going on inside the paddock. "The boys are barrel racing," she explained, jumping from her horse to open the car door for us so we could watch from between the fence posts. We saw one ranch hand after another take their turn riding as fast as they could around a barrel then charge back around another on the other end of the corral. "Barrel racing helps train horses for roping and cutting."

"Yes, I know," Evangelista said in a presumptive tone, as if everyone could tell by looking at her she had won two ribbons in riding competitions herself in her secular life.

We hadn't been watching long when we were interrupted by a cowboy on a horse leading two other horses toward us by the reins. He leaned over and handed each of us a leather strap but stopped when he saw Sr. Evangelista's legs were a "might puny" in the length department and both stirrups would need shortening. He slid off his horse and landed as tall and straight as one of the fence posts. Lifting her up by the elbow, he helped her into the saddle so he could make the necessary adjustments to her stirrups. She gave the lanky cowboy an embarrassed thank you that sounded more like an apology for needing his extra attention, or for being short, I wasn't sure which. Giving us a glance around, he headed off our greenhorn questions from two city slickers by mounting his horse and rode back to the other wranglers.

Gee, I wonder what gave us away, I thought, my worn out garden boots, Sr. Evangelista's veil, or the baggy jeans she was wearing under her habit?

I've always enjoyed riding, I thought, as I guided my foot in the wooden loop of the stirrup and pulled myself up on the horse. But looking down from up here, I had second thoughts about my health. With MS, could I take all the bouncing and off-balanced leaning? Isn't this just asking for a bout of nausea? How much jarring could my head take?

Then I remembered I hadn't experienced any car sickness on the long ride to and from Albuquerque, I felt myself relax, enough to check to see if my antivert (meclizine) pills were still in my jeans, plus the one I'd split in half and kept loose in my T-shirt pocket. Once I felt it was there, I loosened the reins and allowed myself to enjoy the ride…but not for long.

My horse, anxious to keep up with the other two, went into a fast trot. It jaunted up to an edge of a narrow gully and suddenly stopped like it had run into a wall. Trying to see around the horse's head, I saw part of a descent falling away rapidly into a twenty foot drop. Now I knew why Sr. Evangelista had yelled at me to hang on. If my horse was having a hard time deciding whether it could make it, it was another bad sign. I clamped onto the horn with both hands as I heard Sr. Evangelista yell, "Yahoooo!" Too little, too late, the horse lunged over, all I could do was let my arms flail backwards feeling for the cantle on the back of the saddle. I was unbalanced but didn't fall off. Then as quickly as we were at the bottom, I felt momentum carry us up the other side, the horses' massive chest expanding as it heaved forward and we were up the other side in no time.

"That wasn't so hard, was it?" Jane asked, like we had managed to stay a full eight seconds on a bull.

"No, not at all," I yelled back at her, as I waited for my stomach to go back to its normal position.

The gait of our horses was slow now that we were on dry, level ground moving through a mix of dead weeds and parts of tiny purple flowers. A drop of blood, glistening golden brown in the sun, had surfaced on my right wrist where my left thumbnail had dug into it like a trowel when my horse lurched. I wiped the blood on my jeans before it was noticed by anyone.

More dangerous than the sudden plunge into the ditch and bolt up the other side, was the notion I didn't want them to think I couldn't handle what they could. This way of thinking set a dangerous precedent for the rest of my life in wanting to see how far I could push myself, especially with the MS. So I busied myself by trying to maintain the correct riding position by holding the reins unfamiliarly in my left hand, refrained from holding the horn like an amateur, and most of all, I tried not to slump.

Maybe it was listening to the snorting and snuffling of the horses as we clomped through the field, or maybe it was in catching the blinding copper sun in my eyes as I glanced up that sparked the memory, but I recalled another incident involving horses that happened when I was young, and even though I hadn't thought of it in a long time, it was truly an unforgettable memory.

Periodically my father would take us to a race track to bet on horses, and as an alcoholic, probably so he could drink. My mother enjoyed the afternoon outings at the track also; the thundering hooves, the flurry around the track, the thrill of having a horse win, place or show.

I was five or six years old on this particular family outing. The whole family went, but with only a couple of younger siblings born at this point, our brood was considerably less than a crowd.

I was in my mother's reach but on my own to watch the horses with their jockey parade pass me. As a youngster I was captivated by the large animals prancing by, one by one, on the way to the starting gate, some trotting, some whinnying, some bucking, in a completely different world of flowing manes and tails. Looking through the wire fence as the jockeys rode the horses only twenty feet in front of me enabled me to have a close, personal view of each horse. Jockeys were riding them but my focus was entirely on the horses.

During the first race I noticed something on one of the horses. It looked like a fuzziness, not frizzy or fluffy, but a blurred fuzziness around the edges. Tugging at my mother's sleeve, I told her this was the horse that was going to win, and it did.

In the second race as I watched the jockey's prance past me, again I saw one horse emanating a fuzziness. Getting my mother's attention, I assured her this was the horse that was going to win, and it did. (None of the other horses had any shimmering around them).

When the horses were brought onto the track for the third race, again I saw the indistinct fuzziness on the edges on one of the horses. Not only that, maybe because I was so happy I transferred my happy feelings to the *fuzzy* horse because it turned its head and appeared to smile at me. I never actually saw big long yellow teeth, but I *knew* it had given me a broad smile.

I approached my father and told him which horse was going to win and I heard my mother say, "You'd better listen to her, she got the first two right." But my method was not as tried and true as his racing program and he didn't bet on my horse, which won. The three races having depleted his funds, we went home.

Even with time to gain perspective, I am no closer to understanding what happened that day. This awareness of a separate reality was not something I brought on myself and I have never seen it on a horse again. I left the track wondering whether the other horses in the race (if animals are purer than humans in regards to sin), could they see the fuzziness too? And if they did, did they "let" the fuzzy horse win seeing it was favored by God in this way? What did this say about free will?

As I mentally drifted back, I thought again of the dirt kicked up on the track by the horse's hooves as they raced around, the bits of torn hope littering the stands in losing markers tossed aside like used corks out of champagne bottles, and the small whips tucked under the jockey's armpits were all just images to me now.

I wondered at the timing of this memory; had it surfaced because of the geomorphology of New Mexico's rock shapes, starting with the most uncommon one in the vicinity, the Emperor of the Dump? Or did the incredible beauty of New Mexico's land formations cause my internal perceptions to cross over into my external perceptions? I had had no peculiar sensations that day other than a feeling of happiness. Was the horse's pent up energy so ebullient that it wasn't able to contain it in the normal perimeters of its physical body causing it to effervesce over in an outburst of uncontrolled energy?

As I thought back, there wasn't an air of unreality about it at all; it seemed normal and natural. Wasn't everybody seeing this fuzziness around certain horses?

I listened to the creaking sound leather makes from the saddles moving with the horse's frame as I followed Sr. Evangelista with Jane leading the way. In an expression of respect at the strong rays of the sun, I thought, "No one appreciates the sun as the veritable orb it is." The sun's rays acting like a Dream Catcher had caught me and I was in their spell.

The two horsewomen leading the way, their forms silhouetted by the sun, I felt the urge to again look at the source. And even though I knew I shouldn't, I looked directly into the sun. For a time I was without sight, reckless and maimed, my purpose blinded. I wondered if this is what New Mexico does, obstructing one's focus for a time by its beauty so that it can bewilder and enrapture the observer?

As our horses plodded through the broken remains of brush on a beaten down path, I was aware of a pinching sensation on my face from the sun. I knew I had to attribute the timing of the race track memory with the spell-blinding effects of New Mexico's firebrand of the sun. I realized the beauty and euphoria I felt watching the equine racers was similar to the pleasure-giving beauty I felt in the New Mexico's landscape. Enlivened by this realization, I gave a little kick to my horse urging it to keep up with the swishing tail of Evangelista's horse.

I readied myself to receive a guiding motion from the sun, drawing my eyes and mind to again risk another look in its direction. But this time it was driven with a glad eye. This time I let the sun leer at me all it wanted, blushing my face in a rosy glow while I welcomed whole-heartedly New Mexico's deliberate bewitching under the orange red sun in the sky.

Chapter 27—The Pueblo of Zuni

It was not like other Catholic churches, Our Lady of Guadalupe was a historic Mission Church.

Inside the Zuni Indian reservation, the few residences looked very much like those off the reservation with yards and gardens and flowers, and trash cans standing out in back. The homes weren't all bunched together in an urban crowd though, it was not *tract* housing that started out on a city planners' desk. These dwellings were well spaced with an occasional country lane cutting between them. There were no sidewalks, and for that matter, the roads weren't paved either.

No midmorning rush here, no one dashing up the sidewalks or traffic down the roads. A dog walking through the neighborhood looked enquiringly at me probably thought, "just another tourist" and went unperturbed on its way. It was right, I guess I was. I felt I had been given this time alone so I could look around. I liked to be able to "feel" the atmosphere of a place; maybe that was what the dog was doing too.

I pulled open the heavy wooden door and stepped inside the empty Mission. It had the smell of antiquity peculiar to old buildings as I took a few steps on the stone floor toward the pews. Looking to the front at the altar my eyes wandered around the cross, sanctuary, lectern, and over to the pulpit. I let my eyes drift to the right, and with a shock, I saw I had been mistaken; I wasn't alone. Somebody in a supine position up on a scaffolding was quietly painting.

The deliberate motion of the brush as it went from palette to mural, palette to mural, was the only movement inside the Mission. Suddenly I felt self-conscious.

Taking a seat on a pew I didn't know if I should say anything to him. He obviously heard me come in and since he hadn't vocalized a hello, I didn't either. I sat and watched the lone Indian artist work in silence atop his high perch and stopped feeling ill-at-ease as we both of enjoyed the quiet together.

Inside the Mission Church, it was impossible not to feel imbued with history. The heritage of a people was being directly applied to the surface of the adobe wall in a mural of images from past centuries. I could make out little of it from my location beneath him as it ran the length of the church on that side. Curious to see what the wall opposite me looked like, I twisted around and saw how it spoke to the onlooker in wordless outbreaks of voiceless shapes; it had been completed with vivid birdlike religious figures together with the likeness of Catholic saints. How unlike these images were to the Stations of the Cross depicting 14 crucifixes representing the suffering of Jesus typically found in Catholic churches. Interestingly though, these paintings show similarities between Catholicism and Zuni spirituality.

In an abrupt moment of disquiet from the peace inside the Mission, outside I heard the sound of several sets of footsteps briskly making their way to the front door. A man with a deep voice reached the wooden doors first offering to courteously hold the door open for the rest of the staff from St. Francis Retreat, and in walked Srs. Hyacinth, Godwina and Evangelista who had gone to inform the Zuni Visitor Center of our arrival[22] and to greet the priest stationed here. He smiled and waved at me as he walked by.

"*Keshshi* (welcome), Fr. James," we heard from the rafters in recognition as the group shuffled in.

"Thank you," the loosely collared priest called back at him.

"That is Alan," the priest introduced, pointing to him, all of us following the line of his finger through the planks and poles supporting the platform in the mission cum art studio. I noticed the painter was wearing a long T-shirt over trousers without a painting smock. He must be a very careful painter, I thought, glancing again at his unstained white T-shirt. I couldn't help feeling this fastidiousness crossed over to his painting in the attention to detail and was an indication of his character; conscientious, careful, patient.

"Alan has been restoring the 18th century murals," Fr. James told us. "He's devoted years rejuvenating the natural colors and preserving the murals from further atmospheric damage. In here sheltered from the outside, the multi-branched lighting fixtures hanging from the timbers in the roof give off a certain amount of light from the bulbs but he uses mostly natural light for as long as he can before the shadows ease him out, isn't that right? asking the artist."

"It's true, Father," Alan agreed, tilting his head to one side so he could see us, and appealed, "It would be good to tell them why the murals are important." And from his perch above us as we stared up at him, he dipped the end of his brush into paint and added another dab to a wing of the mural.

Happy to share more information about Zuni art, Father motioned with a hand for us to sit on a pew. "The murals are important because they depict kachina dancers representing the four seasons, or Ko'ko' as the Zuni refer to them, in the summer and winter cycles and they use a variety of colors relevant to the individual kachinas.[23] "See for yourselves," Father said, tilting his head toward the finished wall to let the brilliant colors speak for themselves.

"Different tribes have different kachinas," he said, shifting his weight to the other foot. "For example, there is the *Kokopelli* kachina, an ancient Anasazi symbol that provides abundance, fertility and rain. For the Navajo, the *Hemis* kachina brings corn crops to maturity, while the *White Cloud* kachina represents the beauty of the clouds to show the importance of rain; or the *Prayer Eagle* kachina as protector of all, representing power, healing and wisdom; the *White Buffalo Warrior* kachina is seen as the bringer of hope, the *White Bear* kachina is used for protection, wisdom, courage and healing and is believed to possess spiritual strength."[24]

He cleared his throat and continued, "They are different from *fetishes* which are objects carved out of shells and stones and believed to have spiritual powers. Once the object is blessed by the Zuni, it is said it contains the spirit of the animal it represents. Kachinas are important to the nature and essence of what they represent and you'll have no trouble differentiating them from fetishes once you see how ornately kachinas are put together with feathers, pieces of leather, and turquoise."

We sat on the pew grateful to be receiving this lesson in Zuni art.

"We mustn't forget the Zuni Corn Maiden. She typifies the down to earth beliefs buried in the culture's subconscious," and the priest related her story. "It's told the Zuni Maiden walks through corn fields among the new growth blessing the young stalks with abundant water and protection, unfurling them as she walks."[25]

My first impression of the Mission had been one of protection too. It was funny, I remember thinking, the mission looked more like a fort than a church. And if it hadn't been for the wooden cross erected on top, I would have sworn I heard a bugle faintly in the distance. The large rough uneven timbers extending from the plaster and adobe on each side of the Mission gave the impression the walls were well-fortified strongholds ready to defend from any direction. Everything combined, the Mission impressed me as a beautiful work of western architecture and I was glad the murals had an artist who cared enough to match the beauty of the outside with beauty on the inside.

But why was there a solid wall of plaster surrounding the whole Mission? One last barrier from invaders?

Sliding his hand along the back of the pew as he walked Father continued, "The Old Mission Catholic Church was built in 1539 and rebuilt in 1968 when it fell into disrepair due to non-use. Have you heard of the *Seven Cities of Gold*?[26] Well, the Spaniards had. They arrived in 1540 in search of the 'streets that were paved with gold'. Monetary reasons are not always a driving force in a person's life, I knew, and I didn't think greed was pushing the dedicated artist to finish. In restoring the murals, I had the feeling he was really working on helping to restore his people and this was what was driving him. I could imagine him picturing the animal figures from the murals running free over a distant sprawl of green hills thick with woods, wingspans gliding comfortably over brooks, drinking from lakes filled with clean water. If he was, was he also envisioning a peaceful valley in which the creatures on the wall could live forever, like his people. I knew this kind of devotion wasn't spurred on by the incentive of gold.

Noticing Alan changing his position along the wall, father raised his voice and aimed it at the metal perch and asked, "Restoring the murals has almost become a lifetime project for Alan. Isn't that right?"

"A labor of love though, Father," we heard, as the painter began to work in a new area along the mural.

Getting up we followed Father James in between pews and pushed into the center aisle, each of us pausing to genuflect before the tabernacle where the Eucharist is kept, as Catholics do.

He lead us to the back of the church up a dimly lit staircase. I could hear Sr. Hyacinth's nervous laughter on the stairwell above me as we clambered up the squeaking wooden steps, and then the sound of keys jangling at the top of the stairs. With a hard rattle of keys he pushed open a door and natural light came streaming in through the front part of a balcony meeting us with a wave of fresh air. I saw at the far end of the open gallery, Father was holding his arms out like he was displaying a prize. Turning to see what he was showcasing, it was hard for me to believe what I was seeing. Below us in the back of the Mission were graves! So this was what the outside wall was protecting. Discovering this was dramatic, but more striking still was seeing the graveyard was littered with trash! Maybe timing is everything, as they say; while we were standing on the balcony with our mouths open looking down on the graves, we had another surprise. Our confused faces were drawn to a paper bag being slowly lowered from the other side of the wall. It was let go to fall to the ground with a dull thud. It couldn't have been planned any better.

Father seeing our bewildered looks, quickly explained. "For the Zuni this was not a sign of disrespect at all; Zunis believe once a person is dead their spirit is no longer here. And in truth, it isn't, is it?" he asked. We shook our heads letting him know we agreed but I actually think we were trying to shake off our dumbfounded looks.

"I guess you're right," I said, thinking it over.

Father pulled the balcony door closed tight behind us as we made our way down the stairs and back into the church, our eyes gradually adjusting to the dimness.

I didn't notice contrasting feelings before but I felt them strongly now. What a difference between the vital and alive depictions on the murals[27] inside the Mission to the necropolis on the other side. I felt I had gone from birth to death in one afternoon.

I watched the cross on the Mission grow smaller and smaller as we turned left onto the highway heading for Gallup. Twisting around to face forward, I was in my usual position in the back seat looking out on the uneven sweep of desert brush, watching as the speed of our car blurred spiny succulents into indistinct clusters of softness along the way.

The impressions the paintings made, I discovered, were not so easy leave behind. Images of the powerful kachinas dressed in colorful costumes and masks danced through my mind as we drove, and I easily pictured the dancers bounding off rocks, winging up hills, slipping untouched through entangled limbs of cactus.

My thoughts drifted back to the mural painter in his eyrie. He didn't brag about his accomplishment and abilities. He hadn't hung a sign over a beam warning visitors, "Quiet! Artist at work!" He quietly worked by himself not expecting any fanfare. It made me ask, did the artist set the tone for the Mission or did the Mission set the tone for the artist? Both were unpretentious, humble, and modest; the Mission in its simplicity of adobe and wood beams; the artist in his retiring disposition and self-effacing manner.

And even though we saw many souls buried outside the Mission, I realized there was one soul left inside: the indelible soul of the Zuni people painted on the walls of the church.[28]

Chapter 28—Vanity, Vanity…

Was I surprised when my seemingly benign thoughts sparked an unflattering memory, one I had conveniently forgotten. I could feel my face slowly redden as I acknowledged how different my motives were from the Zuni painter. The memory also began with the unmistakable odor of paint…

I knew it was going to be a really hot Arizona day. The sun had already burned off the morning haze leaving the landscape looking baked and cracked, the heat rolling in waves over everything evenly, gulches and hills alike. It was ten thirty in the morning and I had just come up from the garden when the superior asked me to join her in a walk round the back of the monastery. I felt privileged being included in the request because normally Trappistines don't "pal" around together walking and talking.

I followed her along the outside the wing of bedrooms on grass that was either yellow, brown or turning to dirt. As we walked by a tiered clothesline cemented in the middle of the long lot and I waited for her as she picked up a wooden clothes-pin that had dropped off and fastened it back on the line.

Monasteries are generally nondescript by choice. Ours, though, may have been showing a little *too* much of the original character to suit the superior. When we reached the end of the building she stopped and asked, "You see how the wood is showing through the paint in places on the eaves? How would you like to put another coat of paint on the eaves? Do you think you could do it?"

When I first came to the monastery I would answer questions with an honest assessment of the situation. "No, it's not a good time for me to drop off your papers to so-and-so right now." Or, "Maybe after I finish practicing tomorrow's music I'll be able to help you." But after receiving corrections on the matter, it finally sunk in that such questions were not questions at all, but gentle instructions. Not this time though. This was one time the superior actually wanted to know if I could take on such a physically demanding task.

Visually I tried to measure the building from base to top. I knew I could handle it. It was a low building and using a ladder I didn't think would make me feel I was in a high wire act. Directing my eyes to the projecting lower edge of the roof, I told her I didn't think it would be too difficult because the eaves weren't that high, and this was before I knew I had MS "You can?" she repeated, scrunching up her face while looking at the sun. And as I kicked the ground with my garden boot, I was glad to know I wouldn't have to worry about drop cloths.

"Fine," she said. "Only do this section," pointing the length of the back side, which included a corner turn and several rooms beyond. "It gets most of the direct sunlight. Don't push yourself, take breaks, and drink plenty of water."

Way ahead of you, I thought, as I eyed the neatly coiled hose near the edge of the building. I wasn't checking the proximity of water, I was peering into it to see if a snake was coiled inside the coils.

I knew painting was difficult but I was looking forward to having my body stretching upward for a time instead of having it bent over hoeing, weeding or picking.

The next morning instead of heading down the hill to the garden, I went around the side of the building and found a wooden ladder, a gallon of white paint, and a wide bristled brush and roller waiting for me. Now every morning and afternoon work period, I was up on the ladder and soon I had made noticeable headway on the eaves.

Along with my progress I also noticed how much time I spent admiring my work, giving the finished parts many approving looks, rewarding myself ten times over with my own pats on the back.

As time went on I began to notice two other returns for my work; being up on the ladder, full face in the sun, my hair had begun to pick up very blond highlights, and completing the summer look, I developed a brown tan.

To my chagrin, the Novice Mistress, Sr. Diane, had noticed them too. There was not much she could do about the tan, but there was definitely something she could do about my beachcomber hair. One evening after supper, scissors in hand, I was subjected to a session of cutting and snipping starting in front that doubled back and searched for more. By the time she was finished I was lucky if I could pull *any* pieces of hair out from under my veil, blonde or otherwise.

Oh well, I thought, shrugging my shoulders as I looked down at all the dismembered blond pieces lying around my feet on the rug in her office. We aren't supposed to be attached to anything anyway, regretting her mutilations that severed another link to my former life.

To make matters worse, I had all I could to stop the left side of my lip from uncontrollably snarling upward when I passed her now. It was worse when I thought she found joy in targeting the blondest pieces, now picturing them at the rusty bottom of a trash can turning pink.

My lessons in humility weren't over yet. The month had passed, and with the eaves completed, I had gone back to my usual routine of morning work in the garden. It was a few days later when I was in the middle of cutting off some fresh of rhubarb, selecting several of the fleshy leaf-stalks for the kitchen hoping the cook would turn them into pies, I heard the sound of a truck stop at the upper level by the monastery. A discussion of men's voices followed.

Hearing the bells signaling the end of work, I straightened up, gathered my stalks, and trudged up the garden hill to see what all the commotion was about. I was surprised to find the cowboy carpenters had been called in (men hired on occasion to help with the bigger jobs around the monastery).

As I reached the top of the hill, all the rigmarole I was hearing fell into place. The cowboy carpenters had been asked to fit aluminum siding over the eaves protecting the wood even more than all-weather paint could. I knew by the time they had finished all that would be seen of my paint job would be the flash of the sun on the oxide. All my hard work was to be covered.

Miles away from Zuni at this point, we passed a shadowy row of cactus on the other side of the highway, from my seat in the car I was surprised to see how late it had become, late in the day and late in the sense of my ill-timed opportunities for growth. First with the hair, then the eaves. What colors were vanity and pride anyway?

Thinking back to the murals and the decades they have been a work in progress for the painter, I realized there was one thing I had in common with them; I was taking a long time to perfect too. Slumping lower on the car seat, I did the only thing I knew might help restore my sense of self-worth and make me feel better: I promised myself I would *never* breathe a word of this to anyone.

Chapter 29—Jiggity Jig

"God doesn't move the mountain; He gives you the strength and power to climb it."[29]

All week long I kept trying to convince myself I had nothing to worry about concerning the train ride home and subsequent drive back, and now here I was being driven to Gallup's station, forcing me to believe I'd receive the strength to climb this mountain.

My concerns were mainly of the housekeeping type and most of them had to do with my physical ability and well-being: packing my luggage, carrying it to the train, and storing it. Then unloading it, carrying it down steps of the train to my ride which I hoped would be there. But these worries were nothing compared to the anxiety produced knowing that the trip back would involve driving on a lonely desert road by myself for over 13 hours. This brought its own set of problems: "Was that steam coming from the radiator?" "Should I turn off the air-conditioner?" "Is the radiator cap cool enough to touch?'

What had become increasingly clear after having been made aware of the innumerable places of interest to visit within driving distance was that I needed my car. And just as important, after being exposed to the New Mexico's beauty, was to bring my camera back to record my incredible stay in Indian country.

I booked a seat on the train back to Los Angeles from my dwindling resources. I rationalized the expense to myself and to Sister: "We really should have another car at the retreat in case the retreat's breaks down," and, "What if you have to go away unexpectedly like before? This way I won't be stranded again."

So I found myself back on the *Southwest Chief* bound for Los Angeles. It was only going to be a short visit, just long enough to tell my family about the retreat; how the conference room almost glowed red in the twilight, how beautiful the surrounding hillsides were in their barrenness, about how I was staying in a hogan (I'd leave out the bobcat episode though).

All the while assuring them wholeheartedly they would feel much better after my *next* visit because I was definitely bringing my camera back with me and they would be able to see pictures of the places I was describing.

I would assure them, "Certainly I know about visitor etiquette when it comes to Indian cultures." It was the first thing I learned when I arrived in Gallup; never photograph people, places and things without asking permission first. Although common courtesy, here in the southwest it goes deeper then that, when you take a picture, some Indians believe you are taking their soul along with their likeness. I would tell my family this belief held the same significance for the Zuni tribe too, and I already planned to leave my camera behind when I witnessed one of their traditional dances. My hands would be lens free was my plan.

Settling back in the hard black seat for the long ride gave me a lot of time to think. I thought of the quiet way of the Navajo and how drawn I was to their laconic nature, with the Zunis taking a close second, thinking of the steadfast nature of the mural painter. Fortunately the other passengers on the train were mostly Indian and didn't try to engage me in conversation. Just as well too, because with all the swaying and gentle rolling motion of the passenger car I needed to keep track of how I was feeling. After about three hours, I swallowed the half pill of antivert I had in a pocket when I started feeling queasy. It was amazing how this pill did so much.

I remembered these pills had worked on the train ride going *to* Gallup although antivert could make me sleepy. I realized how calming it was just *knowing* I could do something to stop any gathering symptoms of an anxious passenger. More importantly, I realized how much MS seemed to be related to my emotional state. It had become apparent to me now that I could literally make myself sick. But if that were true, I reasoned, my thinking could keep me healthy as well. The problem was, I didn't know how much I could push myself yet, emotionally as well as physically. Riding horses down an incline was one way to stretch my nerves, and unconsciously, I think finding my limitations was a major reason I decided to come to New Mexico and work at the Retreat.

I have always thrived in sunlight; the hotter, the better, which is unusual for a person with MS I didn't worry about that *too* much though. With every person having a different physique, it stands to reason that heat will effect every patient differently.

Heat and MS don't get along. I hesitated when I read this because I have always thrived in sunlight, the hotter the better. It wasn't until my 'big' attack when I was in severe heat and under heavy stress, did I understand that this was a deadly combination for me. Heat doesn't worsen symptoms permanently but it can exacerbate problem areas already effected; even hot baths may worsen symptoms for some people. I have never experienced muscle weakness due only to hot weather without stress. What I wanted to do was create a double blind, setting up a situation where I would eliminate one of the previous factors, either heat or stress.

My year working on top of a hill in New Mexico in the thin air of a high altitude and full sun gave me such a chance. I discovered after the period of a year, I felt fine. Stress tests measure an individuals' heart rate and oxygen intake during strenuous physical exercise, I had measured emotional elements alone by eliminating personal stressors, the very things that got under my skin that only I was aware of. Even though the year had flown by, it felt like a year waiting for the other shoe to drop as I kept track of the movements of my arms and legs conscious of flexibility seeing if anything else on my body weakened. When it didn't, I had to assume stress was more of a threat to my health than heat.

My brief stay at home was overshadowed the entire week by the knowledge I had to drive back through Arizona's Mojave desert by myself; cleaving the Cottonwood Cliffs, scaling the heights of Bill William's Mountain in third (maybe second) gear, directing myself into the unrelenting beauty of the fossilized tree section of the Petrified Forest National Park in eastern Arizona. I was concerned by the heights of the mountain ranges straining my engine as much as I was frightened by the waterless stretches, but the thought of bringing my camera back so I could capture the enchanting beauty of New Mexico compelled me forward like a beam of light.

The key to long distance driving when going it alone, I assured myself, is to *not* to picture what can go wrong with the car; a tire going flat, battery not turning over after every a pit stop, running out of gas, fan belt snapping like an old rubberband. I have my former car to thank for this cautionary practice because the engine on a Beetle looks very much like a lawnmower and it was easy to imagine the worst. It wouldn't take much to disengage the little four cylinder motor; a stick flying up and wedging itself into the flywheel, and suddenly with a stuttering and a puttering, I would be stranded in the heat.

The white Mustang I owned now was more powerful than the air-cooled VW but came with another likely problem, a radiator to overheat. I avoided picturing that too.

The drive to Gallup was about 850 miles, not a bad drive at all. On the map the route looked straightforward enough, head east with only a few convoluted buckles and crook-neck turns to slow a car. I didn't see any dizzying heights that were more fit for llamas than cars, or indications showing the disruption of road closures. And as long as my car was in good working order with all its horses pulling together, I intended on driving straight though. I told myself it was an easy drive, like driving to the mall 15 times, if the mall was 60 miles away, somehow it made the drive feel less threatening; windy weather permitting.

With the radiator filled to the brim, oil and gas topped off, the car was tuned and ready for the long drive. I unscrewed the top of the canteen I had on the seat beside me and checked for the umpteenth time to see if it was full. Confident I wasn't going to die of thirst, I put in a favorite music tape, eased it into gear, and pushed on the throttle.

Choosing a sleek, sparkling semi, I tagged along at a comfortable distance, using its draft to improve my mileage. It wasn't until I was outside the city, adjusting the rear view mirror, that I became aware of the real direction I was traveling——out of the rolling racket of traffic jolting and jerking as it raced along the freeway making me go faster than I wanted to go, away from the smell of diesel fumes and noxious emissions clinging to my nostrils, far from the din of noisy trucks with drivers reciting arrival times like litanies, steering clear of restless lane-changers: I was entering the quiet and calm of the desert with the warmth of the sun on my elbow and the swoop of a hawk in my eyes, both of us welcoming the clean rush of air over our outstretched limbs.

I wasn't surprised when what started as the lone cry of a hawk, turned into the words of Fr. Walchars because I had gone from the spiritual intensity and quiet of the desert to the noisy urbanity of city life, and going back to the desert again felt like I was going on retreat. It was fitting the words of the retreat director should come to me in the voice of the hawk directing once again, *God doesn't move the mountain; he gives you the strength and power to climb it*, and my fears floated away on the wings of the hawk soaring high over the dot of white traveling down the empty gray road alone.

Chapter 30—The Volunteers

Inviting strangers into your life is risky. But that is exactly what Sr. Hyacinth did during the week I was away by enlisting the help of two male volunteers. I knew she had put them through a rigorous screening process but that didn't make me feel any better, because as much as I didn't want to admit it, lonely, quiet places like this *sometimes* attracted individuals who weren't firmly grounded in reality. I was positive the phrase *bona-fide psycho* never once crossed Hyacinth's thoughts.

George and Thompson didn't know each other when they arrived but their motives were the same, they each wanted to volunteer for their church. The fact that St. Francis Center was located on a frontier across from a Navajo reservation opened up a wide range of possibilities beyond peace, quiet, and Indian summers with real Indians. It could be a starting point for excitement and adventure as well. Their choice wasn't hard to understand because this was part of my reasoning too, drawn-in by the cowboy and Indian mystique of the West.

Hyacinth was more of a trusting soul than I. This was due in part to her robust physique; it made it hard not to acquiesce to her wishes. Even now, as her figure stood gracefully before me in black habit and veil, crucifix dangling from her neck, for some reason the unprovoked image of her gently tapping a rolling pin against the palm of her hand comes to mind, although I had never once seen her lose her temper.

I wasn't as jovial as Hyacinth either. Where she was good at hoping and trusting things would work out for the best (I was living proof), I immediately began seriously questioning the motives of the volunteers. I knew that even when references were checked, you never knew which type of personality you were going to get, balanced or unbalanced, and then it might be too late. Were they running from something? If so, what? Was ambition driving them? Guilt? Love? To me they were *onus-probandi*; a blind bargain.

George and Thompson were each assigned to different small hogans; George to *Sister Water* hogan and Thompson, to the *Brother Fire* hogan. And like me, they understood when the retreat needed more bedrooms, they had to welcome retreatants into the extra bedrooms in their hogans during overflows.

They were expected to eat their meals with us in the small dining room, and were shown where the washer and dryer were, in case they had it in their minds volunteer work included maid service. This didn't present a problem for Thompson because he was older and had been out on his own several years, but even after George was shown how these appliances worked, it soon became apparent he seldom bothered to use them.

The volunteers were very different. George was over six feet tall and round-shouldered, and had a small paunch protruding from his belly. He was dark headed and had a line of black freckles running across his cheeks and nose that looked like they had been stenciled on with a fine marking pen. It gave him a whimsical, impish look so even with his Goliath stature, it made him seem friendly and approachable.

Thompson was shorter, about five feet five inches with a massive shock of red hair and a face plastered with red freckles. So many it was impossible to pick out a plain patch of pigment without splotches of red. I caught myself trying to find one but turned away when he caught me staring.

George's personality I was to learn, came through the olfactory, but Thompson's personality came by way of his tongue; yak, yak, yak. I was surprised he considered himself monk material for an Order of silence. Volunteering was to prove himself novitiate-ready: docile and obedient, definite requirements for a monk.

I was surprised, too, by Thompson's English accent, "Ello," he said cautiously, his eyes narrowing as he sized me up, wondering if I would be someone he could get along with. I wondered the same. With a classy accent like this, I pictured him sipping tea with his pinkie in the air, a well-bred gentile, and polished person. I expected him to be well-mannered and polite, avoiding sudden movements and loud speech, just the type to work around self-effacing, quiet Indians. I was glad to have both volunteers join our staff. If nothing else, to show outsiders we weren't alone.

It was my first Sunday back at the retreat after my whirlwind trip home. Sr. Hyacinth took us, Sisters, girls and volunteers (Fr. Lighterman declined) to Gallup to hear Mass said at one of the larger parishes in Gallup. Youthful Ruby, wouldn't settle down, acting as if she was sitting on a red ant hill. Nothing pleased her. Even the 'chatterboxes of birds' sweetly singing in the trees lining the street annoyed her. And when Sr. Celeste fastened the ends of her hat under her chin, she acted like Sister was tightening a noose around her neck.

"*Sacre bleu,*" I heard Sr. Celeste murmur under her breath while steering Ruby into church by the shoulders.

"Shhh," I directed at Ruby softly after noticing a woman's disapproving look as Ruby passed. The little scene ended with Ruby walking away in a huff and I couldn't help feeling what a different calling it is to *want* to work with children. I didn't know how they did it.

We were on time for Mass and straggled into the church already crowded with patrons hoping to hear spiritual and moral encouragement to keep them on the straight and narrow. We couldn't all sit together because we were a large group; the retreat Sisters were ushered into a front pew, Sr. Celeste and her charges were directed to a seat behind them, with George blocking Ruby's escape route if she became fidgety or had the urge to break for freedom.

Ruby could give both Sisters a run for their money. She was always ready for a game of catch-me-if-you-can, so I was relieved to see her finally sitting peacefully on the pew on her best behavior and didn't have to worry about her making another scene; a small reward for good parents or good caretakers.

Thick-wasted Sr. Hyacinth was no match for Ruby who was like a gazelle, quick and agile. Although Hyacinth's athleticism was evident in everyday tasks—directing and controlling a vehicle, rearranging furniture, carrying luggage etc., she was no match for a squiggling child. Hyacinth's face was naturally ruddy anyway but the few times Ruby truly exasperated her, Sister's happy florid face would go bright red; if Hyacinth was a teapot, she'd be whistling hard, bubbling hot over water, and her lid would have blown off. It always ended the same though; a remorseful Ruby would slink up to Hyacinth and apologize, letting Sister know how sorry she was for making her collapse in a chair.

I knew many of the priests in town. Most had conducted or attended retreats, and I knew the priest now saying Mass gave interesting retreats. For the sake of our new volunteers I was glad he was officiating as their introduction to Gallup, this Mass will show them what they could expect during their stay.

Looking past Sr. Hyacinth and company toward the altar, I saw Father swinging a long chain with an antique bronze incense dispenser on the end. He flung it first in one direction, then to and fro in another, doing his utmost to have its burning perfume scent[30] ready as many areas as possible in preparation for Mass. In his final swing, he casually swung the chain towards Hyacinth's group as if he was purifying her entire entourage in one sweep.

And as I watched through a mist of incense and drifting candle smoke settle on the colorfully robed priest, the unnatural faces on the statues, on the shimmer of gold from the tabernacle, it made this religious tableau look as if it had been rubbed from a lamp.

Everything was going along smoothly although the priest was reading the parts of the Mass quickly, like he had an appointment to keep. He was speaking at such a fast pace I stopped trying to read along with him as he zoomed in a blur through the doxologies, devotions, Gospel and communion prayers. He was reading the prayers so rapidly that it must have offended Thompson's idea of the proper way to say Mass. When the our new volunteer couldn't stand it any longer, he stood up and in front of Mary, Jesus, Joseph and God Himself yelled, "What's your hurry? What's more important than Mass? Nowt!"

I am shy and don't like attention. Thompson's shocking outburst brought me out of the ethereal scene straight away. I wanted to disappear into the wooden hymnal holder on the pew in front of me. I was glad I was sitting in back.

With half of the congregation sitting to the front of the church, maybe most of them hadn't heard Thompson's bold comment over the Mass supplications. I was relieved the priest showed no signs of being disturbed by the rude interruption and continued his lickity-split rendition of the Mass. (If he *had* heard, he was controlled enough not to become angry at the verbal affront.)

The congregation was mostly Anglo with a number of Navajo attending too. There may have been other tribes present, but after Thompson's outlash, I wasn't looking around.[31] (For second language Indians, it is probably hard enough trying to understand a regular English accent, but trying to understanding the musical pitch of the Queen's English of Thompson's accent may have been impossible.) What did *nowt* mean anyway?

Two pairs of lively black eyes regarded Thomas and me suspiciously from over the top of the pew in front of us sneaking quick peeps at who had the strange accent, or who had the audacity to yell like that. It wasn't only squirming girls that were curious, adults turned to stare in our general direction too. I was amazed at how fast my body responded to what I thought was threatening, instantly replacing my insides with an unsettling sense of humiliation. I could feel my body tense with every head turn.

Thompson's remarks were uncalled for of course, but what made it worse was his forceful tone. A stentorian voice is usually backed by something; anger, muscle, sometimes lunacy. His shocking outburst reminded me of another shock, and immediately I was back in Arizona at Our Lady of the Desert monastery talking quietly with Reverend Mother Eleanor. It put today in prospective.

I had been a novice for over a year when the Sr. Eleanor asked me out of earshot from the rest of the Sisters to read a letter she received. She wanted to know if I recognized the name of the person who sent it. With rototilling waiting for me in the garden, I was only too happy to make time for the disruption of some light paperwork before I started.

Handing me the letter, I saw it was written on both sides of a sheet of unlined white paper in slanted handwriting, and if I were to guess, I would think it was a woman's script because the cursive strokes were large and flowery. As I read, I was taken by how one thought flowed into the next in an uncontrolled lucidity. But what made the letter confusing, was most of the time the writer didn't bother to use periods so I couldn't tell where one thought ended and another began. I had to read most of the sentences twice to understand what they meant, and even then I still wasn't sure.

Working my way down through the rambling thoughts, I had to admit I had no idea what the writer was talking about. Then I turned the page over and focused in on the signature and my heart almost stopped when I read, Charles Manson.

Somewhere in the distance I heard the voice of Rev. Mother asking, "Well, what do you think? Should I write back?" While I was still staring at the name, I heard the voice again asking, "Should I write back?"

In a very steady voice, I heard myself say, "No, you shouldn't write back." My shocked nerves told me I needed to sit down.

Remembering the letter helped me make extensive attitude changes. By bringing healthier perspectives to the present, it allowed me to see what was *really* important; Ruby's minor scenes of impatience were just that, minor. Come to think of it, she really was well-behaved for her age, especially being a fetal-alcohol-syndrome baby. And she never ran from *me*, not since the day I entrusted her with a few of my *special* hiking tips: remember, keep hands out of pockets to help break falls; walk backwards away from a bobcat while screaming (which she practiced); never run downhill!

I began to see her behavior wasn't dreadful at all, it was almost exemplary for someone dealing with the amount of problems she's had to cope with; born to alcoholic parents which affected her physically and mentally, her mental capacity was stunted, being taken from her chaotic home and placed in a stable one. It hadn't been easy for Ruby. I made it a point to be more tolerant the next time she refused to do something.

And the priest could use any tempo he wants to celebrate the Eucharist. Insisting on anything else would be impatience and intolerance on my part. It's not the momentum of delivery that is important, in fact, portions of the liturgy the priest recites are in a tone audible only to himself. (These parts are known as the *Secret*.) Volume control and speed are not what mattered in the Mass. I was glad the priest didn't try to appease his parishioners 100% of the time; a little verbal blood letting now and then just might be a good thing.

Even Thompson's yelling was no match for the letter. Nothing could compare to the gravity of what Manson's letter represented. Thompson's petulant behavior made me see how trivial it had been and forced me to review my own uneasy reactions and see that the problems were mine, not Thompson's. After my embarrassment subsided, the most disparaging remark I had about the incident was, "So much for the reserve of the English."

As I walked out of the incense haze down the church steps away from the crowd voicing their good-byes, a wave of crisp cool air met me. It was with a combined sense of relief and peace that I thought of the favorable turns I'd undergone in my thinking during Mass and looked down to see my thoughts mirrored in the leaves being turned over as they fluttered along the gutter. Stepping off the curb over them, I realized when the priest had expressly told us to "go in peace," this was one time I actually did.

Chapter 31—Mudheads

The great circle path of the sun in its celestial sphere brought multicolored leaves to the ground in a frosty canopy of living color. It also brought the dancing gods of Zuni.

It was nine o'clock in the morning when Thompson and I set off for the reservation. Regardless of the season, the blue-gray interior in my car was already too hot to touch. With all the windows rolled down we pulled onto the highway and a pleasant windy breeze blew over us during the entire hours' drive through the high desert.

Teddy bear cholla dwindled in number as their thirsty roots reached the pavement of the road, while every scenic sandstone bluff and tall block mesa increased my eagerness to experience a Zuni dance. When I'd heard the dances were prayerful and not just performances, besides looking forward to seeing the authentic Indian dances, I was actually looking more forward to experiencing an awakening of my spirit. Longing began to grow in my heart; even before we even reached the pueblo, I was already moved.

We skirted the perimeter of the 700 square mile Zuni reservation heeding the exhortation from the retreat Sisters encouraging us not to miss this once-in-a-lifetime opportunity to watch the Zuni dance. Not having Hyacinth in charge added more worry to our trip; I was responsible now and it called into question my decision to bring Thompson along. I hoped I could trust him not to yell or make a scene like he did at Mass in Gallup. This was worrying me because at times the unrealistic image of him tied and stretched in the sun would come into mind, along with the phrase mob-mentality. I was aware that violators on a reservation were subject to Tribal laws[32] but I was also aware I was not carrying extra money for bail for Thompson if he needed it.

I decided the best thing was to forestall him by explaining if he ever yelled in church like before, this would be the last time I would ever take him on one of these excursions. I only hoped it sunk in. To drive home my point, I made it as clear as I possibly could, intimating I could always find another willing travel companion. George probably was a good tire changer, I calculated, and I wouldn't have to convert 32 pounds to metric for him either. Maybe one of the Novices would like to come? Reading the thoughtful look on my face, it was as if he read my mind. He convinced me he would never call out his opinion again. I only hoped his solemn word about behaving meant something, especially since I wouldn't be able to turn to Hyacinth and ask, "What are you going to do now, Sister?"

When we reached the pueblo, we pulled onto an empty flat lot and parked on the dirt. It was sunny and hot and quiet, nothing stirred except the flapping of a crow crossing overhead. I recalled when Sr. Hyacinth brought us to see the Mission, she knew where she was going and was able to pull into the interior and park near the church. I, on the other hand, rolled us to a stop on the outskirts, out of the way. Like before, we didn't see a shop or store or commercialization anywhere.

Stretching as we climbed out of the car, we looked around at a few typical stucco houses with window boxes, not the adobe-brick surfaces plastered in mud one might expect to find on a reservation, but we were only in one small area. It felt good to walk so we strolled down an empty lane. We were approached by a smiling Zuni woman wearing a calf length skirt and a blouse and sandals, asking if we needed directions. We told her we were here to see the dances and she said we were headed in the right direction, and pointed us down the road. She had us turn right at the corner and follow the other people walking we would find there. We thanked her, but before she went on her way, she politely warned us cameras and recorders of any kind were not allowed. And turning toward Thompson said, "No applause either please." Must be his loud hair, I thought.

Making the turn we came upon a number of people walking in the road ahead of us. And the more we walked, the more people came and joined us in an unhurried walk down the middle of the unpaved street.

No one spoke, we were all walking in a hushed and purposeful gait. From this point on, because of the silence, things began to feel special to me and took on a spiritual tone, like I was preparing for a meditation. In fact, it felt like we were in a walking meditation and the silence accentuated this feeling. I sensed a definite feeling of camaraderie and a kinship of spirit as we walked along in silence.

In a way this spontaneous procession accentuated the importance of these ceremonies by adding solemnity to the ritual. And as Thompson and I followed the growing swarm, it was as if we were in a spiritual undertow that was dragging us into a different state with the urgency reflected by our faster pace.

We were slowed by a bottleneck caused by a group of people standing around the base of a ladder, but everyone was patient and orderly. Looking up, I saw a woman halfway up on a rung and I watched the woman above her disappear as she went over the ledge to the roof. The group at the bottom was milling around waiting for their turn to climb. Each person made their way up until it was my turn, then Thompson's, and we both scrambled up the large, wooden ladder leaning against the *kiva* (ceremonial lodge) as the entrance for viewing. (The only way to see the dancers was to watch them from the roof of the *kiva*.)

Once we were on top on the flat gravelly surface of the terra-cotta colored building, walking to the other side of the roof, I was surprised we could look down behind a short adobe wall on a spacious enclosed patio that had no floor. Beneath us closed partitions along the walls of the square courtyard had been secured in readiness for the dancers. The whole time people were still climbing the ladder and coming over on the roof to make their way to the other side, searching for the best bird's-eye view they could find. Not knowing what to expect I was startled when somebody yelled, "Here they come!" and two sides of a large solid gate were dragged open, to make way for the arrival of the dancers. One by one, trim and muscular men entered the patio dancing, first one danced by, than another danced in; about thirty painted dancers in all, about twenty yards apart. It took some time before the entire line was finally in the square.

Thompson and I looked at each other. About thirty bare-chested men spread out a few yards apart from each other wearing hideous face masks, their bodies smeared with mud, gyrated and twisted in dance steps evolved out of their own personal movements on the packed-down earth. There was no music, only an individual voice in Zuni dialect would call out at times that made people laugh and sometimes a cry would be let out. And even though the dancers were dancing by themselves in what seemed to be a choreography of their own making, each acted like he was more than just a dancer, as if the interpretive movements meant something else.

Knowing that primitive dancing was usually religious in nature, I tried to find meaning from the bodily movements; could the stamping of feet be an inducement for rain to fall by simulating thunder? Were the cries pleading the powers of nature to protect their crops? Did the duration of the dance influence the corn crop? Did the more they dance mean the more corn they would have? It was fascinating to think about while deriving pleasure at being a witness of the action.

Thompson and I watched captivated along with all the others on the roof, mostly Zuni women. At times a dancer would call out something in Zuni dialect and people would laugh. They leapt and hopped and stomped in the dirt on the square in no particular arrangement of dance routines (that I could determine). It was a remarkable sight to see, even if I felt we were sticking out like sore thumbs; one red headed Anglo and a blonde one, every other person there had black hair. And depending on tourists, it was quite possible Thomson's red hair was their first glimpse of this color. Oddities or not, everyone smiled at us and were friendly and polite.

After a couple of hours, Thompson touched my arm and suggested we go. What he found repetitious was exactly what enthralled me. It reminded me of the monotonous sounds and repetitiousness of chant, and even without understanding what I was hearing and seeing, I could have remained there until the dance was over.

Before we left I took one sweeping look around, down on the spirited dancers in the patio, at the long, black-haired Zuni women on the roof next to us watching their ancestral heritage, and knew I had been presented with one of New Mexico's greatest gifts; the intimate sharing of an ancient prayer.

The sun was high in the sky by now as we climbed down the ladder. Sneaking away as inconspicuously of we could, as I felt for the next rung on the ladder with my right foot, I couldn't help thinking of the words from a poem by St. John of the Cross, "…I went forth without being observed, my house being now at rest. In darkness and secure, by the secret ladder, disguised—oh, happy chance!"[33] In climbing down the ladder I had the sensation that little by little I was climbing out of my subconscious, like being roused from sleep. Jumping off the last rung, I hit the ground with a start, fully aware.

"It was worth the climb, wasn't it?" I asked Thompson.

"Smashing! I say, how did you like those costumes? Most peculiar indeed, wouldn't you say with the mud and all? Why do you suppose they muddied themselves like that?"

"I don't know. I was surprised too, mud instead of feathers and paint like I had imagined. This is one dance you could never imagine."

We started walking back on the deserted road until we were halfway back to the car when we met an Indian woman about sixty woman named Linda wearing a silver bracelet and earrings, a rose colored skirt, and sandals. I commented on her hair clips and she invited us into her home to see her collection which she sold. Thompson glanced at me just as I glanced at him, I knew what he was thinking, 'what a stroke of luck to be invited inside a Zuni home!'

Except for her work table off to the side of the livingroom, the inside looked very much like the houses I was brought up in; couch, coffee table, dining table, dishes draining on a rack next to the sink. While Thompson kept Linda busy answering his questions, I picked out three hand-beaded barrettes I liked that were orange and black and white.

Dropping into chairs beside her, we sat while Linda explained about the dance. The weird Mudhead masks show what happens when relatives marry and serve of a warning against incestuous relationships. Mudheads or Koyemshi, are clowns and this dance is the most frequent. The Dancers start in a nearby river bed and dance the entire way to the Kiva. She said the dancing lasts until dawn. Other dances include the Sword Swallowers, the Summer Rain-Dance, the Doll Dance, the Shalako, and Leaving the Gods.[34]

I thanked her from both of us in Zuni, *elahkwa* , for sharing the information and for her time. I told her every time I wore one of her barrettes I would think of the Mudheads and remember the excellent day I spent at pueblo of Zuni.

We walked back to the car in a subdued temper thinking of the day, opened the car doors, climbed in and readied ourselves for the hours ride north to Gallup in the dark.

From this distance it looked like a hologram. Red, yellow, blue and white lights suspended in mid-air on the left side of the road ahead. We were closer to Gallup than Zuni at this point and driving in the filtering shadows of dusk. "I don't remember passing a gas station," Thompson said scratching his head.

"Neither do I. It looks like a man throwing a lasso. Could be a general store."

"Nah. We didn't pass a store either. Might be one of those makeshift shrines people put up when someone dies in a car crash."

With the design of lights fast approaching, it came clearly into view and we knew we were both wrong. "Blimey, it's a pub!" Thompson exclaimed, letting his excitement bubble over like the foam from a beer. In the daylight even with its neon business lights on, we hadn't noticed it on the way out. He followed his statement with the realistic fact of how thirsty he was. He didn't have to convince me though, the last water we drank was at home, besides I was curious to see what the inside of a real saloon looked like.

As we pulled into the Dry Gulch Saloon's parking lot among a number of pick-up trucks, I wondered how safe my car would be displaying California license plates. And to be on the safe side, I gave Thompson a cautionary warning before we went in, "For heaven's sake, don't make anybody mad!"

"Not to worry" I heard the words trailing behind him as he headed for the door.

The Dry Gulch didn't have butterfly-wing doors we could push open like in Westerns, but it did have every conceivable insect known to the Southwest stuck in its screen door. That was something you didn't see every day, as the recently attached bugs glistened red, green, yellow, and blue from the neon sign.

When we walked in, one by one heads turned to see who the strangers were coming in off the desert. No one said a thing. I was disappointed there wasn't a player piano belting out *She'll be coming around the mountain,* but there was a juke-box in the back of the room playing a Willie Nelson song. This was one time I wished someone would turn *up* the country music.

We made our way unobtrusively across the room through the sawdust on the floor and sat at a low round wooden table. The large room was smoky and dim and had rough knotty-pine walls holding in the dirty air, and I could see a couple of men seated at the bar, Anglos, one wearing a tan cowboy hat tilted forward, no Indians[35] though. A few ranch hands seated behind little round tables, sat nursing their beers, filled the rest of the room, and one gent sitting way in the back coughing, put me in mind of Doc Holliday.

We didn't get a "What's your poison?" but we did get, "What'll ya have, partners?" in a gruff voice.

Thompson looked at me and I mouthed the word beer. He turned toward the bar and called, "We'll have two pints please."

Well, now everybody knew he wasn't from around these parts.

The bartender, a big burly man about fifty, responded with "Two pints of what?"

"Why, lager of course," Thompson said smiling.

I added, "We'll have two beers please."

I watched as the taverner pulled back on the spigot and filled two tilted glasses underneath with golden draft. Placing them in front of us, he said, "That'll be three bucks." Whereby Thompson handed him a five dollar bill and told him to keep the change. From then on, we had a very attentive bar-keep who exchanged our empties with frothing full ones without our asking.

The saloon didn't have the long horns of a steer stretched decoratively over the fireplace adding to a western atmosphere, but it did have the owner's long-haired black and white cat stretching sleepily at the end of the bar.

I tried to keep up with the drinking pace Thompson set but after a certain amount, beer just doesn't taste good to me anymore, so I quit. (Thompson didn't know I had MS and it felt good acting like there was nothing wrong). I kept him company while he continued in his rowdydow, which wasn't so much rowdy as it was continuous drinking. When he excused himself, I took the opportunity to duck my head under the wooden table to see if he was pouring his beers out into the sawdust because with all he consumed, he didn't show any signs of inebriation whatsoever, no hiccups, burps, slurring of speech or any unsteadiness about his person. Feeling the floor which my hand, I let the small particles sift through my fingertips as I felt around in the sawdust; completely dry! I had to concede, I was no match for this Englishman and began wondering if there wasn't some truth to the general idea that certain groups of people can or can't hold their liquor. Living proof was draining another glass of the golden liquid down his throat that very moment.

The cat had long since vacated its spot on the counter in the late hour and we decided to do the same. We waited for the country-western song to finish before we got up and left, Thompson earning a respectful nod as we passed from the barkeep. Heading into the blackness outside, we swatted our way through powdery millers, hairy moths, shiny flying beetles and everything else swarming the lighted entrance.

When we had taken a few steps in the cool smokeless air, I motioned for Thompson to stop so we could inhale the strong scent of the sweet desert sage brought on by nightfall, pointing out to him, "This is one of the best parts about living in the desert," if it hadn't occurred to him already.

I was relieved to see my car still in the lot and we climbed in. Trying to see through an unsplattered section of the windshield, I headed the car in the direction of Gallup and leaned back against my seat to watch the lights of the tavern blacken in the rearview mirror. As we pulled farther and farther away until there was only darkness behind us and darkness in front of us, all of a sudden I felt comforted Thompson was in the car beside me.

On one level I was listening to someone happily feeling their alcohol, explain the differences between pubs in England and bars in the States; how pubs at home were not only for drinking but for having a meal as well, when he started describing an example of a typical pub meal consisting of potatoes, cabbage, bacon and sausage…on another level I was thinking about our day, reviewing all that had happened: climbing the ladder to the roof, waiting and watching for the dancers to arrive, the nature of the pig masks, the welcomeness of Linda. And feeling around in my pocket, pulled out a barrette. Turning it over in my fingers, I again felt a gratefulness for the hospitality of the Zuni by allowing us to glimpse into their wonderfully mysterious world.

Thompson continuing to describe his favorite meal with gusto, Thompson went on, "…and a plateful of scones and wedges of Wensleydale cheese…"

But my thoughts were far from food. Topping off the day, I could hardly believe we had visited a real, live, western saloon.

Announcing the rest of a toothsome meal like he was selecting items off a cart, "…with jam to top it all off, you couldn't ask for anything better," licking his lips.

"Exactly!" I said in firm agreement, while imagining the Mudheads continuing to dance in the dark, perhaps now around flaming ends of torches…

On a dark night, kindled in love with yearnings—oh happy chance! I went forth without being observed, my house being now at rest. In darkness and secure, by the secret ladder, disguised—oh, happy chance! In darkness and concealment, my house being now at rest. In the happy night, in secret when none saw me, nor I beheld aught, without light or guide, save that which burned in my heart. This light guided me more surely than the light of noonday, to the place where he (well I knew who) was awaiting me, a place where none appeared. Oh, night that guided me, Oh, night more lovely than the dawn, oh night that joined Beloved with lover, Lover transformed in the Beloved! Upon my flowery breast, kept wholly for himself alone, there he stayed sleeping, and I caressed him, and the fanning of the cedars made a breeze. The breeze blew from the turret as I parted his locks; with his gentle hand he wounded my neck and caused all my senses to be suspended. I remained, lost in oblivion; my face I reclined on the Beloved. All ceased and I abandon myself, leaving my cares forgotten among the lilies.

Ascent of Mount Carmel, St. John of the Cross.
Image Books, Garden City, New York 1958.

Chapter 32—No Bull

It didn't look much like a show-bull. What a shock it was to drive in and see this enormous animal, big as a buffalo, lumbering through the retreat yard no matter what its standing was in a 4-H Club. The knotweed embedded in its scruffy black hide gave it the unkempt look of a wild animal and I found it impossible to believe suede could be produced from any part of its rough skin.

From the safe distance inside my car, I noticed this descendant of the once great herds of the American West had pieces of dried weeds and jagged leaves stuck in its stringy tail as well. The fact that it wasn't a pet made my situation worse; would it charge if I were to sprint to the retreat door? Did I want to risk being gored by its two thick horns while fumbling for door keys? I knew as fast as I could scramble, the bull might be faster and I didn't want to take that chance. I was stranded.

After a while, I began to *will* it away. Focusing my attention, I aimed my concentrated thoughts on a patch of brown lawn hoping the animal would pick up my brain waves and look at the paltry growth in which it had to choose from, *become dissatisfied, regret its decision* of choosing to graze here, and *wander away*. But as hard as I thought, it never even glanced at the brown patch. I must have weak brain waves, I decided, and went back to regular thinking.

The afternoon shadows were growing longer and longer as I waited in the car watching the beast move over the gravel paths cropping the ends of grass and weeds with its yellow teeth, its snuffling displayed in undignified bits of pink gravel stuck to its wet black nose making it look like a piece of confectionery candy was stuck to it.

Sitting in the car I realized how I had brought this stand-off on myself. Now that the volunteers were here I had extra time and the idea came to me to take classes at the university. Sr. Hyacinth was all for it, so I registered for education classes at the campus, which brought me the predicament I was in now. Returning from class, George and Thompson were nowhere to be found, the Sisters were probably at the group home, and Fr. Lighterman may have gone fishing while working on Sunday's sermon.

Waiting for help gave me time to think, mainly about whether this animal keeping me from my studies was a sign. Was going back to school the right thing for me? If it was, wouldn't God have cleared the way for me instead of sending this living obstruction? Decisions concerning school have to be made quickly because of deadlines, and for a person like myself who hadn't decided on a career path, the pressure to commit can cause a lot of worry, enough for me to begin wondering if the bull was a sign, the equivalent of a ton of bricks.

Although bulls don't have the four-compartmented stomachs of a cow in which its cud is forced back for re-chewing, it still reminded me of my own situation. Wasn't I doing a similar thing by returning to school again? Hadn't I already paid my share of tuition, listened to enough lectures and crammed for enough tests, especially if retreat work was my calling after all?

To be on the safe side, I decided to continue taking classes as a backup because 'man being no better than brute', I worried I might *become dissatisfied, regret choosing this career path*, and *wander away* too. From then on, whenever I convinced myself I needed more academia, the picture of the snorting and grunting mass of brawn in the form of the dissatisfied black bull crossed my mind, and became my bete noire in more ways than one.

No sooner had I come to this decision, I heard the sound of tires crushing rocks on its way up the road to the retreat. Finally! The calvary was here in the form of Sr. Hyacinth. I stepped out by the side of my car and frantically pointed toward the bull hoping she would defend herself. I yelled to her in warning, "You'd better stay in the car!"

I could see her puzzled face crinkling in a "You've got to be kidding" look. Sizing up the situation, she disregarded the forewarning from somebody she thought was probably afraid to say boo to a goose and drove in close, got out of the car with a halfhearted groan and a threatening flick of her wrist, and stood challengingly holding her ground in a menacing stare.

The beast did not like this new turn of events for anything that brazen might have something to back it up with. Disturbed by its sudden lack of force with its own position, and frightened by this bold interruption in its peaceful afternoon of nibbling, the animal turned and made its way between the hogans, escaping down the hill trying to get as far away from Hyacinth as it could. The last I saw, it was hightailing it away from the big, bad sinister Sister, making tracks toward the reservation looking over its shoulder, its swishing tail tucked safely between its legs.

Feeling a flush of embarrassment, I watched red-faced from behind the impenetrable protective metal covering of my car as the animal was shooed away without incident.

Chapter 33—Realm of the Apache

People pass through Gallup on the way to somewhere else which is a shame because the town has a life and a charm all its own. Good and bad, the experiences here were very different from anything I had in my past, from the BIA (Bureau of Indian Affairs) serving many different groups and exerting their influence among the diversity of people living here, to the opportunity of seeing time-wizened faces and distinctive dress of the Native Americans coming in off reservations for supplies.

Gallup deserves more than a cursory look, I thought, as I steered my car through the light morning traffic in downtown Gallup. Thompson, with the pleading eyes of a beagle expressed how much he wanted to come with me. We both couldn't resist the opportunity of seeing Apache country. Especially after hearing Fr. Clark's emphatic invitation, "You must visit!" at dinner one night during a retreat.

That's when the imploring eyes of Thompson began in earnest. The truth was, he didn't have to give me the 'please don't leave me behind looks', I wouldn't have gone by myself. Arrangements were made, we were packed up and out, ready for another road trip looking forward to seeing Fr. Clark's mission operation in Apache country, if only for a weekend.

As I moved over the worn-out white lines on the road to the right lane, different experiences came back to me I had encountered here, from the novelty of using drive-thru grocery windows, to smelling the peculiar odor at health care centers after a delousing, or the helpless feeling I had learning some families were unable to afford $350 for a wood stove for their hogans, and lamenting distressing accounts of Indians passing out in the snow and freezing to death during winter.

Pieces of these scenes faded in and out of my mind like the faded window displays we were passing on the way to the freeway. They made me realize just how many unusual and striking moments, I, as an outsider was lucky enough to experience. I still find it hard to believe I have seen so many of New Mexico's wonders and know I will always carry a deep affection for its way of life with me always.

Add to these experiences the surprising fact there are approximately 200 millionaires living here![36]

Gallup is unique—geographically, spiritually, and financially! I recalled the day when all three of these aspects were illustrated at once as I relived the day for Thompson while I drove.

"It was mid day and I was visiting the Navajo reservation with missionary, Sr. Carol. Part of her job was checking on families to see if they had enough food and wood and she wanted to check on a family she hadn't seen for over a month. As we drove deeper on the reservation, I remembered seeing two very curious shapes in the distance that only wind, water and time could have formed. Sculpted like weird rock creatures on the surrounding plain, one was a pillar of rock standing straight and tall soaring cloud-topt at an incredible height in the sky, and next to it was this massive butte, hulking and expansive from top to bottom. The forms made me question how nature could shape two such completely different formations right next to each other, especially when they both rose up (or melted down into) the same dry dusty patch of ground.

Sr. Carol rolled her Bronco to a stop near the family domicile toward a small group of people outside. I had a strange sensation of driving into a living gallery depicting Navajo life; Roberta the grandmother was in the center of the activity, and two younger women at her sides were assisting her, learning as they watched the matriarch.

The grandmother was sitting in front of a large wooden loom made from sturdy tree branches, alternately working a stick over and under strands of yarn; a red, yellow and blue design already completed hanging around the borders along with tassels set at each corner. She turned towards us to see who her visitors were and gave us both a smile when she recognized Sr. Carol.

The family scene made me feel as though I had stumbled into a Godly place. From the feeling of peace I felt there, I had the impression the family was not only finishing a rug, they were putting finishing touches on stages of perfection as well—patience, tolerance or perseverance. Their lifestyle may seem boring to outsiders (like the routine of a monastery) but when the good that comes from it is known, it becomes admirable, not wearisome.

The oldest daughter sitting in close on a blanket was working a small hand-held implement winding yarn onto a holder, turning out yarn for her grandmother to use. A younger granddaughter with her knees folded under her, was resting comfortably in the shade of a canvas covering protected from the noonday sun. When I mentioned I liked color combinations in the rug, the grandmother's face broke into a thousand pieces. "It will bring a good price," she told us, still smiling.

"Eventually it did," I told Thompson. "Months later I learned from Sr. Carol the rug had sold for hundreds of dollars. Looking back, if I had a choice which scene I would photograph, the dramatic scenery or the family united working the loom together, I would be hard-pressed to choose one to line up for a picture. Both were inspiring."

My heart beat faster as I approached the onramp to the freeway on a course heading for Apache country to the north. As far as I knew, I had never met an Apache before, so all my preconceived ideas had been formed by television and movies. The only lasting trait I remembered about their entire tribe was that they were good trackers. They could trail over shallow water, double-backs, catwalks, tree branches, even ropeways, yet they themselves were trackless. We agreed this gave them an immateriality.

As my car rumbled farther north, Thompson and I noticed the landscape beginning to change, as if to accommodate the unearthly quality in our thinking. Leaving cactus, tumbleweeds and scrub bush behind, we found ourselves driving between steep-sided oblong mountains towering dangerously high on both sides of the highway. Most of the vegetation now was long wiry weeds sticking out from between the rocks.

I wasn't sure if our conversation was unnerving us or the severe look of the country, but we both recognized a shift in our moods. For the rest of the trip we had a feeling of apprehension and it was easy to imagine Apaches climbing on the rocky ledges as lookouts to warn the rest of the tribe intruders were approaching. It crossed our minds that maybe the spirits of the famous Apaches Cochise and Geronimo were putting a scare into us. In the effort to restore our original sightseeing calm, I told Thompson most Native Americans believe spiritual power was everywhere, but this did little to reassure him. Me neither. If anything, it increased our paranoia.

Unlike any solid rock mass I remember seeing, the stratified rockery lining the road looked like it was made of sheets of black onyx mixed with layers of white quartz. The tiers reminded me of how I used to drip wet sand from a bucket at the beach to build layer upon layer making a tree out of heaped up wet mud. Instead of mud, here nature dropped black and white chunks of flat rocks on top of each other, stacked so high it looked like we were driving through towering cathedrals. Mile after mile of them, they made our passage feel ominous, but we drove on undeterred in the shade of their rugged magnificence.

The hours passed slowly on the road but eventually we reached Fr. Clark's turn off at dusk. I pulled in the parkway, turned off the engine, and we sat for a moment listening to the awesome quiet disturbed only by the creaking of the parts of the engine coming to a rest. I would have liked to let my body come to a rest as well after driving for so long, but it wasn't long before a building door opened and Father Clark emerged. He was wearing the casual clothing of an off duty priest in a white shirt, black slacks and button up sweater. We climbed from the car into the cool evening air and stood next to his tall frame. His combed brown hair moved in his vigorous handshake in greeting and I could tell he was a happy person from the laugh-lines scattered around his eyes.

He was delighted to see us and I had the feeling we were an enlivened change being stationed here by himself. Our all-day journey, he thought, was a trivial matter, one he had made it many times himself. (It would have been too, except for my having to wonder the entire trip how my body would react to the drive, like having a slow leak in a tire and seeing if would become flat or hold up.)

We got out and stretched and after a walk around the car to give it (and myself) a quick assessment, I was pleased to see the tires were still up and my limbs were working. I had the usual tension in my shoulders from being in the same position for a long time behind a steering wheel and the soreness that comes from sitting for hours in a bucket seat.

"Wasn't the scenery spectacular?" Fr. Clark asked proudly, as he led us through a low front yard gate to the rectory.

"Yes, it's really beautiful," I agreed, keeping to myself how I found the unusual rock precipices visually threatening.

We talked for an hour sitting in the scarcity of a room devoid of knickknacks, trinkets and remembrances common in secular households.

"You must be ravenous after the drive. I saved you a little something," motioning us to the dining room through the kitchen. Like the living room, the kitchen was practical, not cluttered, other than a few postcards and notes held by magnets on the refrigerator.

Over a dinner of fish, baked potatoes and green beans he had waiting for us in the oven, I remembered this is the same Friday meal we would be having at the retreat. It was funny, but listening to Fr. Clark describe the benefits of volunteering in Apache country, it became clear how much I preferred to work in desert surroundings where I could see for miles under the radiant light of the sun.

We listened to Father's idea about volunteering for a year or two. I knew it wasn't for me but noticed Thompson thinking purposefully about it. After all, he was in a different country, he should try to see as much as he could. I knew how volunteers are subject to the vagaries of superiors, directors, managers, or administrators; not to mention how weather could shut a place down. So I was all for Thompson keeping Apache country as a backup. Using Fr. Clark as a lifeline was smart. I would have done it myself if I hadn't been wasn't already very pleased with my situation at St. Francis.

The fact that we couldn't stop yawning did not go unnoticed by Fr. Clark who walked us to a guest house and our respective bedrooms. Saying good night, he turned off the hall light and went back across the patio and into the kitchen. I could hear the clinking of plates and silverware as he washed the dinner dishes by hand.

More than ready for a good night's sleep, I couldn't wait for my muscles to relax and just plain rest after the all the driving. Vivid thoughts of the imposing massif loomed even larger in my mind when I closed my eyes for sleep so I pulled the covers over my head like an impenetrable shield to keep the image away from me. It wasn't until I rolled over and faced the window that my keyed up thoughts were replaced by the steady crooning of crickets that finally lulled me to sleep.

The next day my muscles were weary but rested. I felt no numbness on my face (or anywhere) and my vision was holding steady, I knew it was going to be a good day, no matter what. Thompson and I planned to start the day by attending Fr. Clark's morning Mass, so after a quick breakfast by ourselves, (Father up early and out) we headed out.

We walked to a small unpretentious Catholic church down the block and joined the few parishioners in a town smaller than Gallup that were willing to get up on a Saturday morning; regulars comprised of a few older women, one couple, and a couple men.

In the time when most businesses closed on the weekend, there was literally not much to see. Thompson and I strolled up one side of a single street and down the other side admiring the window displays of Indian art and crafts, stopping on a bench under a tree to write the postcards Father left for us in our rooms. The town was quiet and peaceful and I could see why Fr. Clark was taken with it.

The big event for us today would be meeting Father at the only diner open in town for lunch. At 12:00 we met at *High Feathers* diner where Father was waiting for us outside in his good Mass clothes, shined shoes and white collar. He led us into the small diner that had a portion of a counter in the back and eight small square tables with laminated plastic white tops and flecks of gold in the padded seats. I was struck by how *'50s* it looked even way out there.

We studied the menus and ordered three hamburgers and three chocolate malteds from a clean shaven middle-aged cook taking down our order on a pad. There were a few other customers around us, all Indians, I could tell by their beautiful long straight black hair and high cheekbones. I had the impression because of their ages, 15–25, this was the local hangout except for one fact, adolescents are usually loud and boisterous, these weren't. There was no horsing around or loud music blasting out top forty hits. They weren't whispering, they were speaking softly.

Finishing our lunch in between Thompson's elevated sputtering, it seemed like the more food he consumed the louder he became. He was really into his subject now, presenting a convincing argument why Fr. Clark would do well to take him on as a volunteer in the future. It was when Thompson dropped his spoon on the table after consuming the last of his malted that Father and I knew the dessert was like adding fuel to a fire because of the sugar rush. His enthusiastic conversation grew in decibels, so much so, I had to wait for his pitch to drop before I could cut in and ask Father an obvious question, "Why is everyone else in the diner so quiet?"

Quietly he said, "That is the way of the Apache." Father said in a low tone, "They feel loud speech is rude and is a sign of bad manners."

Thompson taken aback, laid his right palm flat on the table and pivoted around on his arm sizing up the diner's Indian clientele as though seeing it for the first time. "I say, is that right?" voicing his doubts in a somewhat lower tone, admitting he hadn't noticed their low tone until then.

Some people who, after initially lowering their voice, can't remember to keep it turned down. Thompson was one of these people. Out of habit, his exuberant personality had increased the timbre again and rose to the same loud pitch.

Speaking pianissimo, I said, "The life of an Indian has always appealed to me and now I know why, stillness is a part of their makeup; they are true contemplatives."

I breathed a sigh of relief when we left the confines of the diner and our words were lost in the open air. Although I was embarrassed by what Apaches would deem discourteous behavior on our part, I walked away with a privileged feeling of learning an obscure bit of information concerning their manner, one I'd never read as a footnote in a book about the Southwest.

As the three of us walked on the sidewalk to father's house I realized how up and down the state of New Mexico, from the family of patient rug weavers I watched outside of Gallup, to the silent customers in the diner in Apache country, to all the isolated Indians living in remote areas on reservations, I was convinced the spiritual energy so easily felt in New Mexico is due to the peaceful lives of these individuals. A quiet presence spreads gentleness over the rolling hills. Enduring patience extends tolerance across empty plains. Selfless efforts flood spirituality to overlapping on banks. Peaceful and humble spirits imbue shapes of nature with anthropic stature. And combined, they enrapture land with blessings.

After the months of listening to Thompson talk, the sound of his voice was now like listening to a cat purring; it was a sign he was happy and content. I was used to it. The question was whether Fr. Clark had the same congenial response toward this facet of the Englishman's personality as I did, or did he view Thompson's lingual dexterity as a disability.

Strolling leisurely along the quiet stretch of road to the rectory, Father and I were pressed into hearing the Englishman's recruitment campaign that would allow him to work as a volunteer[37] here in the future. His oral crusade sounded like a pamphlet for vocations and I flashed back on all the religious promotional material I'd received at one time or another, volunteer programs included. Invariably, the organization in question would send a brochure containing a picture of a bright-eyed woman about twenty-two usually wearing glasses, all smiles because she'd made the right decision, her face scrubbed so clean I could make out where the washcloth had scrapped off the membranous tissue on her face leaving only innocence and purity shining through. And in the background, a statue of a female saint.

For the male branch of religious, I sincerely doubted they would send Thompson a brochure featuring a picture of a opinionated youth still cutting his eye teeth, trying to settle down, standing open-mouthed, hoarse, thumping a fist on a desk, expounding on one thing or another, trying to get a point across while engaged in an endless argument; a podium standing off to the side.

I noticed Fr. Clark walking along quietly let a few remarks from Thompson go unanswered, unchallenged. Was he deciding whether Thompson had the special qualities needed to volunteer here weighing the pros and cons too, like I was? Non-stop talking was a big con. It all came down to words with Thompson; first calling out at Mass in Gallup, now the loudness of his regular speaking voice. Here, where a soft voice is a necessity, I really didn't think Father had any other choice but to say no but one never knows.

By the time we reached the gate to the yard of the parsonage, Father was tugging thoughtfully at his collar. Finally, with a serious face, he let us hear his thoughts. "You know, Thompson, controlling people with words is another way of getting your own way."

The enormity of this statement must have hit Thompson like Chief Seattle's spear because instead of a rebuttal, Thompson stood very still and replied, "You know, you're right Father." With those words, Father swung the gate open and we walked through.

During our trip to Apache country Thompson came away with a contact person and back-up plan if he should ever need one; Fr. Clark tentatively got a hard working volunteer when the time was right; and I saw the great beauty of a area that turned out to be one of the most mystical and transforming regions this side of the Pecos River. It had to have been, Thompson didn't say much all the way home.

Chapter 34—The Brothers

The crowd of Brothers piled out of their mud splattered station wagon in the Retreat yard and parked next to the statue of Jesus. It was a dramatic entrance as car doors opened and the Brothers of Charity, dignified and grand, graced the yard. The six religious were wearing long dark blue cassocks with matching soft brimless blue caps and large crucifixes swung freely from around their necks.

I watched as each one stepped from the large automobile into a sloppy mixture of ice, mud and dirt that had turned to slush and each habit was immediately dragged through the partially melted snow, everyone's but Brother Drake's. In an instant he had gathered handfuls of his blue material and stuffed the excess in his belt holding up his slacks underneath and was standing off to the side pulling at a loose thread from his shoulder. The long habits of the others had picked up a brown line of demarcation around the bottom edges, but the forward thinking of Bro. Drake kept his hem unspoiled, clean and dry.

The Brothers lived in community in a residential section of Gallup where they taught and tutored at the elementary schools in town and on the Reservation too. Their ministry was teaching but they were also involved in charitable works as well. A few times when the Retreat had an extra large group of retreatants, after a call from Hyacinth, the Brothers would show up and help with parking, move tables, cook, serve, and even pitched in to with the dishes. Generally they showed up on Friday and Saturday nights to help with the biggest meals. Working alongside us in their long garments, because their footwear was hidden from view, I felt like I was working with a group of Russian dancers on skates, zooming this way and that, doing the work with panache.

Brothers Jeremiah and Drake attended the University like I did so I saw them in passing. Jeremiah ran a 12-Step program in a gym at a local high school and was quite talkative and outgoing. Bro. Drake was more introspective and reserved. The Sisters and I looked forward to having all the Brothers show up for KP because of their jovial good-natures; plus they were a big help.

During our Advent retreat, Pam, a regular retreatant, offered to help in the kitchen, as retreatants sometimes do. When Pam suggested felling a fresh tree for the retreat dining room as a gift to St. Francis Retreat, Bro. Drake and I jumped at the chance to go. After her donation was approved by Sr. Hyacinth, we prepared to go in search of the perfect Christmas tree in the surrounding mountains for the dining room.

In the winter wonderland scenario in my mind, I saw Pam's invitation as the adventurous undertaking I have always wanted to go on; trudging through pristine untracked snow, selecting a perfectly shaped fir, carefully cutting it down, dragging it back to the car while a light dusting of snow fluttered from the sky. A flake sticking to my eyelash was evidence we had chosen the right evergreen and we should look no further.

This was my fantasy. Actually, driving half way up the nearest mountain in a forest thick with pines, we found the trees always looked better on the other side of the hill so our search took us well out of the way. Enjoying the search, we settled on a large fir, the perfect large size for a large dining room. The single woody self-supporting stem unbranched some distance from the ground really was the most perfect tree. We took turns sawing and flopped it into the bed of the truck, being careful not to bend its weighty limbs backwards. We drove homeward with the strong scent of pine in the cab and sap sticking to our hands.

Our trailblazing ended though, when Pam driving her truck, could feel the traction give way on the ice-packed tires. We lurched, we spun, we jolted, and slid. And to our astonishment we gradually started sliding sideways down into a ditch off the road.

Stunned, we sat afraid to move as we waited for the truck to come to a complete stop. Glancing over at the passenger window, I saw a solid wall of white as we pushed against the snow, packing it against the mountain. With our right shoulders jammed together, the Mazda finally came to a rest. No one moved. Breaking the tension, Pam repeated the short catchy ad jingle, "Mazda, we are DRIVEN!" and we burst out laughing.

Unraveling our limbs from each other, we scrambled out one at a time and stood in the snow and waited on the icy road. With our teeth chattering in the cold, a farmer finally came moseying down the road riding a tractor. Seeing Brother Drake, dirty and disheveled now, hailing him to stop, the old-timer kindly offered to help. Hitching a chain to the Mazda's bumper, the strong engine of the farm tractor strained and groaned but hauled the truck back up to the road. Wishing him a chorus of "Merry Christmases," we went on our way expressing our profound thanks over and over as we drove away.

Back at the Retreat, Sr. Hyacinth was glad to see we had picked out such a large tree and taught us the country way to stabilize it instead of using a metal holder with screws to wind into the bark. She had us hoist the tree into a plastic gallon container which we filled with large heavy rocks. We secured it by piling on more rocks. I was surprised when it actually worked.

That evening we ended by stringing lights and popcorn, hanging bulbs, and laying strips of glittering tinsel on the branches. With the fire crackling sap from the firewood, we sat on the couch with our feet stretched to the fire sipping homemade eggnog, admiring the decorated tree.

The next day I read in the local newspaper that twenty-three people had been ticketed for cutting down trees over the weekend without permits, and I wondered what with all the commotion we had made, how did they ever miss us?

Retreatants enjoyed the tree well into January, but permit or no permit, my Paul Bunyan days were over.

Chapter 35—Canyon de Chelley

We advanced on the edge of the overlook with dread.

Canyon de Chelley (pronounced Shā) takes the hiker back millions of years but stepping a few feet forward could lead a person straight into the world to come. Being a part of the girls' Navajo heritage, the Sisters thought it educational in a variety of ways to bring them for a visit; a good outing for all of us, Sisters, girls, and volunteers.

Located in northeast Arizona, covering 83,840 acres on a Navajo reservation, the national monument was established 1931 and has 26 miles of sheer sandstone cliffs ranging to more than a thousand feet in height. Indian culture dating as far back as 350 A.D. to 1,300 A.D. may be seen inside natural crevices in the walls along with the ruins of prehistoric cliff dwellings and pictographs. I learned the spectacular red sandstone cliffs were a backdrop for hundreds of Anasazi ruins which may be seen by taking self-guided tours.

This is the other Grand Canyon, and as far as I was concerned, the better of the two because it wasn't overrun with tourists. I didn't see any restaurants or shops so maybe that's why. I learned there was a tourist center close by which offered details and maps to frequented sites of White House Pueblo, Mummy Cave and Canyon del Muerto but we didn't see the center either.

This was how the spectacular reddish brown cliffs should be seen, at one's own uninterrupted pace, by soaking in the breathtaking rock formations, the colors, and the quiet. I could only imagine what the peace must feel like at the bottom of the canyon surrounded by thick solid walls of smooth stone. Luckily we had the place to ourselves, or that's what I thought.

From on top of the canyon, our group stood admiring the dark streaks of deposits on the canyon walls. It didn't matter to me knowing if they were formed of oxide or manganese. They were visually stunning.

I found it interesting that bits of pottery and tools were found on the floor of the canyon from the Anasazi Indians known as the 'Ancient People'. And looking down on the river flowing between large full-grown Cottonwood trees instead of cactus, it was easy to visualize herds of goats and wagons passing along with an entire community living and working there.

So could George. In a last ditch effort before we climbed back in the car and truck for the long drive back, to work off some of his restlessness, he told us he wanted to communicate in some way with the canyon below us, to let it know we appreciated the history and the beauty of Canyon de Chelley.

I will always remember standing high above the wind blown canyon and hearing George's voice echoing off its walls his loud Indian cry of, "Oh, oh, oh, oh, oh, oh, oh, oh, oh, oh, oh," as he thumped his mouth with his fingertips and seeing a habitue making himself known by walking out from under a group of golden poplars to a clearing, looking up, and giving us a prolonged wave!

Chapter 36—Away We Go!

My feet have never been colder! But it was worth it. From my ankles to my toes, it felt like I was walking on solid blocks of ice in the shape of feet, even with the thick gray woolen socks Sr. Godwina's mother had loaned me. Unfortunately, I don't think I got any sleep despite her concerned gesture.

I had been invited to witness an *arpeggio in flight*, as Sr. Godwina's father Stan had described it. And because he felt the expression of musical works and lyrical styles was broadening, Haydn being his favorite, Sr. Godwina had been raised in a home where classical music was played throughout, so his musical statement would mean something to her. I had to wait till the weekend was over before I could flip through a dictionary passed 'aroma', 'around', 'arouse' before finding arpeggio. *Arpeggio, a chord whose notes are sounded in quick succession rather than simultaneously.* And when I learned the meaning, it made perfect sense. This was how the hot air balloons go up, quickly but not all at once, changing the sky into a magnificent chord of color, a silent melody heard differently by each onlooker just by lifting their eyes to the sky. It made spending a night in the traveling igloo worth it.

I thought back to the day before. With winter on the horizon and the days getting shorter, we'd pulled into Cutter's Field during the night. Stan was driving us in a large blue camper pulling a smaller silver trailer behind him. Godwina's mother Josephine, acting as navigator, was sitting in front beside her husband with a map spread across her legs pointing the way as we moved along. From the numerous open camp fires emblazoning the flat fields around us, many others were willing to brave the cold to see the start of the Albuquerque Balloon Festival like we were.

Not from this part of the country, I didn't know what I was in store for and I looked around trying to absorb as much as I could. The dark sky cloaked in black enclosed the expanse of this temporary encampment like a lid covering a pot keeping in the cold air, while dim lights plotted the fields identifying human lairs. I watched our headlights bounce about lighting up the few pedestrians making their way over the packed down field of dirt. They were not tarrying, but walking with the purpose of getting out of the cold. This was a field trampled by people's goings and comings; rutted by foot traffic and had given way to dead brown weeds mashed into the dirt that were momentarily highlighted as we drove through. No wind blew across here as if it too was holding back waiting till after tomorrow's spectacle.

Stan maneuvered the camper around trailers, campsites, and even tents, bumping his way over fields flattened by spectators and enthusiasts that had settled in for longer than a weekend, if propped up bikes and makeshift clotheslines were an indication. I saw people bundled up in layers standing as close as they could get to fires, some with drinks in hand while puffing hot breath on the fingers of their other hand. Quick bursts of exhaled breath drifted frostily away as expectation hung as thick as icicles on the nippy air.

I remember climbing into the silver trailer and settling in my sleeping bag with my pulled socks tightly around my ankles and waited for sleep. Using my arm as a pillow, I waited and waited. I couldn't tell whether my cold feet were keeping me awake or if it was the excited energy of the impending liftoff charging me up. The night consisted of briskly rubbing my feet with my hands, or moving my legs against each other like kindling trying to start a fire.

It must have been three in the morning by now. I lifted my head and listened. All was quiet. Trailer doors had been latched and tent openings zipped; everyone was sleeping. Everyone but me. For hours I couldn't buy a dream.

My thoughts wandered around and around filling in the time before dawn, back to the hot air balloon that went astray over the monastery in Arizona with me trying to remember what the intense heat of the desert felt like hoping thoughts of sunburns would warm my body. It didn't work, my feet were still cold as icebergs.

A myriad of loosely connected thoughts floated through mind; how unsafe the earliest balloons were because they often carried a brazier, a metal container holding coals and charcoal to replenish the supply continuously, and on top, a large valve was used for releasing gas controlled by a cord.... I wondered how St. Francis Retreat was getting along without Sr. Godwina and me. Were Tony and George being helpful even though they had to put in double work along with Sr. Evangelista?...I wondered if George, encouraged by the response he received at Canyon de Chelley, would attempt to use his vocal gymnastics of loud monosyllabic tones when a retreat is in session.... I wondered if Sr. Hyacinth would give Thompson another opportunity to cook after his first breakfast fiasco when he cracked open thirty eggs into a pot of boiling water and called it scrambled eggs. I didn't think she would.... And I wondered if this freezing night would bring on an episode of MS.

As I turned over to relieve the weight on my hips, with a sinking feeling I realized I had hit the benchmark moment for all sleepless people, when crickets, insects and other creatures cease their calls and their silence is replaced by thin tendrils of cold air caressing the face like bony fingers. It only means one thing—*dawn*. And riding in on its breeze was the fatiguing reminder I had been awake all night.

And as if a signal had been given by an unseen muezzin proclaiming the hour for prayer, suddenly hundreds of people were up, wide awake, and babbling unintelligible chatter to each other. It was incredible. One moment, all was peaceful, the next, not exactly chaos, but close to it. When the sun came up, everyone put on their coats and gloves and bolted into action. The teams of balloonists knew the air was now the right temperature for the balloons to be inflated, and the mad scramble was on! Literally hundreds of people across the lightening darkness appeared, balloonists, crew members and onlookers offering help.

It meant I had to get up too. Putting on my coat and knit ski hat, I was out the door standing bleary eyed in the hazy semi-darkness with Sr. Godwina and her parents watching people scurrying every-which-way. That's when we heard the first gush of hot air being propelled into an open section at the bottom of a balloon. I recognized the sound from the downed balloon in Arizona and it was fascinating to see at close range (within several feet) what was causing the sound—the rush of air, now hot after forced through flames, directed into each balloon as they lay deflated and stretched out all over the fields like discarded coats at a party.

I was amazed to be able to stand as close as I was to a gigantic red balloon watching the air being blown into it, next to the action. I watched as partially inflated balloons flopped and struggled like wounded animals and lightly bump other balloons when fully they inflated. The balloonists, proud of their balloons, offered rides in exchange for help and to be part of their team. Many spectators accepted and the rest of us would watch and wave as they eventually ventured off on the rides of their lives! This may be what attracts so many people; the chance to go sailing off in the wild blue yonder.

It was alive: multicolored stripes changing color as they went around the whole of a balloon, patriotic balloons praising America in red white and blue, larger than life cartoon characters, and patterns just depicting colorful designs. They made me forget the cold.

In time, scores of full-blown balloons rose before our eyes, incredibly huge and colorful, and like magic, one was a foot off the ground, then two more; all across the field, gondolas defying the pull of gravity by hovering in the air, each takeoff lifting my spirit with a feeling of exhilaration and astonishment. At times balloons blanked out the new morning sun with their deep purples, bright yellows, and soft violets standing against the deep blue awakening sky. Balloons of brilliance in the October azure sky.

High above, the far off whooshing sound of the blowers was intermittent as less hot air was needed, while the spectators on the field added more wood to their fires preparing for the long wait till touchdowns, some close, others miles away. The mood of the bystanders settled into a helpless state of expectation and uneasiness as they worried about friends and family soaring thousands of feet in the air without ropes, guide-wires or nets. The sharp snapping and clicking of cameras was everywhere.

Afterwards with Sr. Godwina and her parents, we sat down to a pancake breakfast, compliments of Josephine in the warmth of their camper, and excitedly exchanged stories about what we had seen during the thrilling spectacular. We described in detail to one another what our favorite snapshot was going to look like when it was developed, discussing bragging rights over seconds. We were in complete agreement though, about how useful a fish-eye lens would have been in covering about 180' at a time.

Cupping my hands around my mug of hot coffee, I was reminded of the previous night of shivering and how I had stepped from the cold trailer the next morning, the first thing I did was exercise my ankles unobserved, moving them up and down and around, wiggling my toes. I relived the relief I felt when I realized the freezing night hadn't hampered my flexibility.

Amazed again how resilient my body is, even with MS, I had discovered that even when I treated it roughly at times (working in the heat of Gallup, enduring long tedious car rides, drinking alcohol occasionally, treating it like it was a Popsicle), I gained confidence I could avoid another debilitating MS episode. I knew the disease acted differently in every individual, so maybe it was wishful thinking on my part, but coming to the balloon festival made me realize I could soar above it all too. I could travel. I could live. I could experience. Like the balloons, living would be limitless and I wondered where my travels would take me too.

Sitting across from Stan I thought, "You were wrong." The bold send-off of the balloons with their flying colors sailing loose and free wasn't an arpeggio, wasn't just a chord of notes at all, it was a symphony! Brilliant colors flying higher and farther away on a motionless drift in front of the soft blue of the sky was an enchanted symphony: New Mexico's grandest finale.

Endnotes

[1] To help with life transitions some Retreat Centers offer discernment retreats to help with the readjustment process.

[2] See Elisabeth Kubler-Ross, *On Death and Dying*, 1969. Also *Living With Death and Dying*, Elizabeth-Kubler Ross, 1981, Macmillan Publishing Co., Inc.

[3] Fetal Alcohol Syndrome is a complex of birth defects including cardiac or neural abnormalities and physical and mental retardation, occurring in an infant as a result of excessive alcohol consumption by the mother during pregnancy.(*American Heritage College Dictionary,* 1993.)

[4] *Yah et-te.* Donald and Ruth Herbert, p. 23.

[5] *St. Jerome and the Lion,* retold by Margaret Hodges, 1991.

[6] *Multiple Sclerosis, the Ultimate User Friendly Guide*, Rocky Mountain Multiple Sclerosis Center Guild, 1999, p.53.

[7] *The Three Days of Darkness*, Louis Barta Publications, 1989. 1996, Cranston, R.I.

[8] From the Moody Blues album: *Days of Future Passed;* "*Late Lament.*"

[9] For more information, see *I'm Not Crazy, I'm Just Not You*, Roger Pearman & Sarah Albritton, 1997.

[10] For more information see: *True To Type,* William Jeffries, 1991.

[11] *Navajo Code Talkers,* p. 52, Nathan Aaseng.

[12] For more information, see *Navajo Code Talkers,* Nathan Asseng, 1992.

[13] Doppler effect: if the source of a sound of a constant pitch is moving toward an observer, the sound seems higher in pitch, while if the source of a sound is moving away it seems lower. The change in pitch can be heard by an observer... (Funk & Wagnalls Standard Reference Encyclopedia).

[14] For more information see *The Gunpowder Plot, World Book Online Reference Center,* May 2005.

[15] Justice, prudence, fortitude, and temperance.

[16] A mystical Navajo formation, near the town of Kayenta, that looks like thousands of babies either laughing or crying, depending which way the imagination is stretched.

[17] Shiprock: a volcanic rock formation pushed upwards by three volcanic pressure ridges in a column over 7,000 feet high in the shape of a bird and is known to the Navajo as "rock with wings."

[18] Because trances were so important to the Native American shaman, the title *powah,* literally meaning "one who has visions," was accorded him.... The word whose spelling was eventually settled in English a *powwow* was also used as the name for ceremonies and councils, probably because of the shaman's important role in both. (*The American Heritage College Dictionary,* 1993.)

[19] Some Navajos believe individuals bestowed with supernatural powers are able to diagnose a person's health problem and restore them to harmony.

[20] Albuquerque-Road Runner Food Bank—(505) 242–2052. Los Angeles—(877) NO HUNGER.

[21] Luminarias are related to *las posadas,* the ritual in which the search by Mary and Joseph for an inn is reenacted during the nights before Christmas with the candles illuminating their path.

[22] Zuni Pueblo asks visitors to check-in with the Visitor Center; (505) 782–4481.

[23] Any of the numerous deified ancestral spirits of the Pueblo peoples; a masked dancer believed to embody a spirit during a religious ceremony; a carved doll in the costume of a particular spirit. *The American Heritage College Dictionary. 1993*

[24] For more on Kachina art see *Southwest Indian Foundation Catalogue,* Autumn 2003 - Issue No. 3, Gallup, New Mexico.

[25] *Southwest Indian Foundation* catalogue, 2002. (505) 863–1037 p.10.

[26] *Francisco Coronado in Search of the Seven Cities of Gold,* Steven Otfinoski. Benchmark Books, 2003.

[27] To learn more about the murals, log on to "Old Zuni Mission."

[28] The current Tribal Council cancelled the lease with the Catholic parish on the building since it hasn't been used by them for over 10 years and hopes to have the Mission be administered by the Tourism Office.

[29] *The Position of Religion in our Modern Society*, 1990, Fr. John Walchars, S.J.

[30] Substances used in incense may include cascarilla bark, camphor, musk, cloves, saffron, sandalwood, gums and spices, balsam, cinnamon, star anise, or the dark red pieces from the dragon's blood plant.

[31] During my limited stay, I found Indians closely resemble other Indians; Navajo, Zuni, Acoma, Hopi, Laguna. For me, it was hard to distinguish one tribe from another.

[32] Zuni is a sovereign, self-governed nation with its own government, courts, and police force with a population of over 10,000.

[33] *Ascent of Mount Carmel*, St. John of the Cross; p.93.

[34] *Dancing Gods*, Edna Fergusson, pages 72-113.

[35] There has always been a prohibition against the sale and possession of alcohol on reservations, however there isn't a blanket law prohibiting Indians from drinking establishments.

[36] *2001 Visitors Directory;* www.gallupnm.org.

[37] Contact Volunteers of America (800) 559-5458, or the nearest diocese for Catholic programs.

Additional Reading

Yah-et-te. Donald and Ruth Herbert. 2000, XLIBRIS.

Giving Sorrow Words. Candy Lightner and Nancy Hathaway. Warner Books, Inc. 1990.

Living With Death and Dying. Elisabeth Kubler-Ross. Macmillan Publishing Co., Inc. 1981.

The THREE DAYS OF DARKNESS. Louis W. Barta Publications, Cranston, RI, 1996.

I'm Not Crazy, I'm Just Not You. Roger Pearman & Sarah Albritton. Davis-Black Publishing, 1997.

True To Type. William C. Jeffries. Hampton Roads Publishing Company Inc., 1991.

Navajo Code Talkers. Nathan Aasend. Walker Publishing Company, Inc., 2002.

New Mexico's Best. Richard Mahler. Fulcrum Publishing, Golden, Colorado. 1996.

Francisco Coronado in Search of the Seven Cities of Gold, Steven Otfinoski. Benchmark Books, 2003.

To learn more about the murals, log on to "Old Zuni Mission."

Zuni Katchinas, Forty-Seventh Annual Report of the Bureau of American Ethnology to the Secretary of the Smithsonian-Institution 1929-1930, Ruth Bunzel. The Rio Grand Press, Inc., Glorietta, New Mexico, 1932.

Katchinas of the Zuni, Barton Wright. Northland Press, Flagstaff, Arizona, 1985.

Dancing Gods, Indian Ceremonials of New Mexico and Arizona. Erna Ferguson, The University of New Mexico Press, Albuquerque, New Mexico 1966.

America Indian Grandmothers, Traditions and Transitions. Marjorie M. Schweitser, The University of New Mexico Press, Albuquerque, New Mexico 1999.

Canyon de Chelley, the story behind the scenery. Charles Supplee and Douglas and Barbara Anderson. K.C. Publications, Las Vegas, Nevada 1971.

(301) 695-1707

Printed in the United States
51102LVS00003B/34-39